A SHORT TEXTBOOK OF CLINICAL PHYSIOLOGY

To My Father

A Short Textbook

of

Clinical Physiology.

PETER F. BINNION

M.A., B.M. (Oxon.), M.Sc. (Med.), Ph.D.
(Queen's Ontario), M.R.C.P. (Edin.)

*Senior Lecturer in Physiology, The Queen's University, Belfast,
and Consultant in Physiology to the
Northern Ireland Hospitals' Authority*

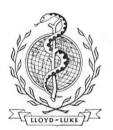

LLOYD-LUKE (MEDICAL BOOKS) LTD
49, NEWMAN STREET
LONDON
1969

PRINTED AND BOUND IN ENGLAND BY
THE WHITEFRIARS PRESS LTD
LONDON AND TONBRIDGE
SBN 85324 078 7

PREFACE

THIS book is an attempt to correlate physiology and clinical medicine, presenting only the essential facts in the briefest possible manner. It is hoped that the text will appeal to those who have completed their entire physiology course and have some knowledge of clinical medicine, hence I make no apologies for omitting much explanation and the reader is advised to consult the larger standard textbooks where necessary.

It is difficult to avoid undue bias towards either physiology or medicine, and it is realised that it is impossible to satisfy everyone with such a book. For this reason it is hoped that readers with constructive criticisms will write to the author so that the book may be made more useful with time.

PETER F. BINNION

Belfast, *June* 1969

ACKNOWLEDGEMENTS

I WOULD like to express my appreciation to the following who have assisted in correcting mistakes and have mentioned important omissions from the text of the original manuscript. Professor I. C. Roddie, Dr. W. F. M. Wallace of the Department of Physiology, Queen's University, Dr. P. Gaskell, Department of Physiology, University of Manitoba, Winnipeg, Dr. A. H. G. Love of the Department of Medicine, Dr. A. McC. Connell of the Department of Surgery, Queen's University, Dr. Mary McGeown, Dr. J. McEvoy and Dr. L. J. Hurwitz of the Belfast City Hospital and Dr. Henry Burger, Prince Henry's Hospital, Melbourne.

In the chapter on the kidney permission has kindly been given for reproduction of diagrams taken from *Physiology of the Kidney and Body Fluids* (Figs. 7–15; 2nd edition, 1968, Year Book Medical Publishers Inc.) and *Federation Proceedings* (1948) **7,** 418, Fig. 8, both being the work of Professor Robert F. Pitts. Miss Margaret Wilkinson typed and retyped the manuscript with great patience and forebearance and Mr. M. Beattie and Mr. Howard Greenaway drew the diagrams for me; to them my debt is great.

CONTENTS

PREFACE v

ACKNOWLEDGEMENTS vi

I THE CELL 1

II THE ENDOCRINE ORGANS 10

III CARDIOVASCULAR SYSTEM 31

IV pH, FLUID AND ELECTROLYTE BALANCE . . 57

V BLOOD 67

VI RESPIRATION 86

VII THE GASTRO-INTESTINAL TRACT . . . 101

VIII LIVER 115

IX THE KIDNEY 122

X THE NERVOUS SYSTEM 138

XI MUSCLE 183

XII BODY METABOLISM AND TEMPERATURE CONTROL . 189

REFERENCES 196

INDEX 198

Chapter I

THE CELL

CYTOPLASM AND CYTOPLASMIC INCLUSIONS

Mitochondria.—They contain enzymes for the Krebs or tri-carboxylic acid cycles (see below) and the cristae of the mitochondria favour spatial organisation of these enzymes.

Golgi apparatus—possible function is to synthesise certain specialised products of the cell.

Inclusion bodies are collections of virus material seen in virus-infected cells, e.g. Negri bodies in cytoplasm of neurones of hippocampus in rabies, Guarnieri body in vaccinia-infected cell.

Ribosomes are small particles (about the size of poliomyelitis virus) on which proteins are manufactured by the cell. They appear to be the reading mechanism for the correct synthesis of new protein material by the cell. A copy of the DNA of the genetic material in the nucleus is made in the form of messenger-RNA (m-RNA). The messenger-RNA moves to the cytoplasm and attaches to a number of ribosomes, forming a complex called *polysomes*. Smaller RNA molecules called s-RNA are also present in the cell and these can bind with specific amino-acids and link these amino-acids to specific regions of the messenger-RNA in the polysome. The amino-acids are then joined together by peptide bonds and released as protein from the ribosome.

The main genetic material is DNA (deoxyribonucleic acid), and RNA (ribonucleic acid) is the other form of nucleic acid present in nature. DNA is formed of a long chain of phosphate-sugar-phosphate-sugar groups and to each sugar is attached a base (four kinds of bases, adenine, guanine, cytosine, thymine are present in DNA). The main difference between RNA and DNA is that sugar of RNA is ribose (deoxyribose in DNA) while RNA contains uracil instead of thymine. Each DNA molecule or gene is specified by a specific sequence of the four bases.

Messenger-RNA contains the bases adenine, cytosine,

guanine and uracil, and a sequence of three of these bases (a triplet) appears to be the genetic code (codon) for the insertion of one amino-acid into the protein chain being synthesised by the ribosome. This process relates the sequences of amino-acids in protein to the sequence of bases in DNA. Proteins are the catalysts (enzymes) used by all living cells and they also fulfil a structural role, hence their production is a basic essential function of a living cell. The way in which they are produced is summarised in the diagram below:

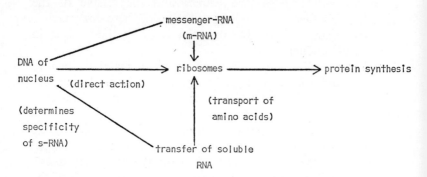

Within the genetic mechanism of a cell (the genome) there are two sorts of genes (i.e. sequences of nucleotides in strands of DNA):

(a) structural genes—sequence of nucleotides determines the amino-acid in sequence in a protein;

(b) operational genes—not clearly understood; control the timing, sequence and other logistic aspects of the expression of genetic potentiality in the cell.

NUCLEUS

DNA is the main material forming the genes which confer certain characteristics on the organism. When the cell divides in mitosis to produce two daughter cells the genetic material is carried on the chromosomes and equally divided between the two daughter cells.

In man there are 46 (23 pairs) of chromosomes classified on morphological grounds by their relative length and centromere position (the Denver system), and numbered 1–22 (autosomes) with No. 23 being the sex chromosome (X or Y). In the gonads in the first cell division the chromosome number is halved (meiosis) so that each secondary spermatocyte or oocyte contains only 23 chromosomes; at fertilisation the full complement of 46 is restored.

CHROMOSOMAL ABNORMALITIES

If there is a failure of a chromosome pair to separate (*non-disjunction*) at the reduction-division (meiosis), one daughter cell will contain 22 chromosomes and the other 24, and the zygote formed by fertilisation will contain either 45 or 47 chromosomes. The chromosomes may break at meiosis and either a piece may be lost (*deletion*) or else incorrect reformation of the fragments may occur (*translocation*).

Sex Chromosome Abnormalities

(i) *One X chromosome only (XO):* Turner's syndrome characterised by sexual infantilism, webbing of the neck, cubitus valgus and usually dwarfism.

(ii) *XXY chromosomes:* Klinefelter's syndrome; males with small azoospermic testes, eunuchoid build, gynaecomastia and high urinary gonadotrophins.

(iii) *XXX genotype:* "super female"; secondary amenorrhoea and subnormal mental state.

Autosomal Chromosomal Abnormalities

(i) *Three No. 21 chromosomes* (trisomy 21): Down's syndrome or mongolism; characteristic appearance of mentally defective individual. This may be due to non-disjunction of No. 21 chromosome or translocation of No. 21 chromosome to become attached to another chromosome (e.g. No. 15; hence total 46 chromosomes but really trisomic for No. 21).

(ii) *Other autosomal trisomy syndromes.* Trisomy for No. 18 (trisomy E) noted in mentally defective child with small mouth and mandibular hypoplasia, low set ears, ventricular septal defect. Trisomy for No. 15 (trisomy D) with mental retardation and a number of other malformations.

There are a large number of diseases produced by either recessive or dominant genes, and in a number of the diseases due to autosomal recessive genes an enzyme defect has been demonstrated. A few specific examples only can be given here:

Diseases Inherited in Recessive Fashion

Enzyme deficiency

Glycogen storage disease	Brancher or debrancher enzyme (see Chapter VIII). Glucose-6-phosphatase. Muscle or liver phosphorylase.
Phenylketonuria	Phenylalanine hydroxylase (for conversion of phenylalanine to tyrosine).
Galactosaemia	Galactose-1-phosphate uridyl transferase (required to convert galactose to glucose).
Alcaptonuria	Homogentisic acid oxidase.
Albinism	Tyrosinase (deficiency in the melanocytes of the skin).
Cystic fibrosis of the pancreas	The commonest autosomal recessive condition in Britain today.

Sometimes diseases with recessive inheritance are sex-linked (carried on the X-chromosome), e.g. haemophilia, pseudohypertrophic muscular dystrophy.

Diseases Inherited in Dominant Manner

Gastro-intestinal tract	Peutz-Jegher's syndrome; familial polyposis of colon.
Circulatory and haemopoietic systems	Hereditary haemorrhagic telangiectasia; hereditary spherocytosis; sickle-cell anaemia; acute intermittent porphyria.
Skeletal system and skin	Osteogenesis imperfecta; Marfan's syndrome; neurofibromatosis; Ehlers-Danlos syndrome; dystrophia myotonica.
Renal	Polycystic kidneys; renal tubular acidosis; vasopressin-resistant diabetes insipidus.
Central nervous system	Huntingdon's chorea; tuberose sclerosis.

METABOLISM OF THE CELL

As mentioned previously, the mitochondria contain the enzymes for the tricarboxylic acid cycle, and it is pertinent to state here how cells, and hence the body, obtain their energy from various circulating metabolites. The metabolism of carbohydrates is summarised below:

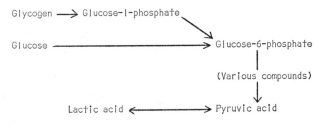

THE EMBDEN-MEYERHOF (ANAEROBIC OR GLYCOLYTIC) PATHWAY

The above pathway requires no oxygen (i.e. anaerobic). Usually pyruvic acid is oxidised to acetyl-CoA (acetyl coenzyme A) and lipothiamide pyrophosphate (from thiamine, vitamin B_1; see Chapter XII) is necessary for this reaction. The acetyl-CoA is oxidised in the tricarboxylic acid (Krebs) cycle to carbon dioxide and water with the energy produced during these reactions being stored in the high-energy phosphate bonds of ATP (adenosine triphosphate—this compound supplies the energy for biological reactions) and note how much more effective is aerobic metabolism, using the Krebs cycle, compared with anaerobic glycolysis with regard to the amount of ATP produced. One glucosyl unit of glycogen metabolised anaerobically to lactic acid yields three molecules ATP while one glucosyl unit of glycogen metabolised aerobically to CO_2 and water yields 30 molecules ATP. The Krebs cycle is summarised below:

Acetyl-CoA + oxaloacetic acid → citryl-CoA
→ via oxalosuccinic, ketoglutaric and succinic acids back to oxaloacetic

The oxidations of the Krebs cycle (i.e. oxidation of the acetyl group of acetyl-CoA) are done through the mitochondrial transfer chain with the production of ATP. Oxidation is affected by removal of hydrogen atoms (by specific enzymes called dehydrogenases) which are then transferred to a series of oxidation-reduction systems arranged as an integral chain in the cell mitochondria. The major part of biological oxidation goes via this system which is summarised below:

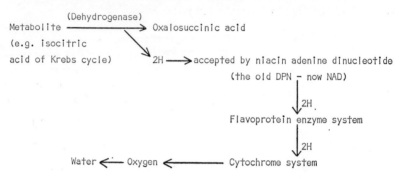

This system is called the *"electron transport chain"*.

Interesting points about this transfer chain are that niacin adenine dinucleotide requires the B vitamin, niacin, and the flavoproteins need riboflavin (vitamin B_2) for their formation (see Chapter XII). Another feature is that cyanide inactivates some of the cytochromes and causes rapid death due to blocking cell respiration.

Fatty acids are metabolised by being degraded to 2-carbon units (acetyl-CoA) (a process known as β-oxidation) and these then go through the above pathways. Unlike carbohydrate and fat, the body has little or no capacity to store protein above that required for normal tissue formation and repair. The metabolism of amino-acids produced from protein in excess of normal body requirements involves deamination (either oxidative or non-oxidative) and formation of the corresponding keto acids which can then be metabolised through the above pathways (excess amino groups form urea).

Interplay of Carbohydrate and Fat Metabolism

There are three pathways for the metabolism of carbohydrate:

  (i) glycolysis;
  (ii) the tricarboxylic acid cycle;
  (iii) the pentose phosphate shunt (not considered above).

These pathways are regulated by alteration of enzyme activity by substances produced during the specific metabolic pathway —*allosteric effects* (a form of feed-back inhibition) e.g.:

$$\text{pyruvate} \xrightarrow{\text{(pyruvate dehydrogenase)}} \text{acetyl-CoA}$$ (the activity of pyruvate dehydrogenase is inhibited as acetyl-CoA accumulates).

The metabolism of fatty acids requires their degradation to acetyl-CoA as mentioned above, and hence fatty acid metabolism can suppress the activity of pyruvate dehydrogenase and therefore the metabolism of carbohydrates, i.e. there is a constant interplay between the metabolism of carbohydrates and fatty acids as demonstrated by the disordered state of diabetic ketosis.

Oxidative Phosphorylation

The above processes are concerned with the oxidation of foodstuffs, and the energy produced is stored in the form of the energy-rich ATP (note: adenosine *triphosphate* has considerable chemical energy in the phosphate bonds). These two processes, oxidation and phosphorylation, are tightly linked or coupled in the cell (*oxidative phosphorylation*), but may be uncoupled by ionising radiations, thyroxine (see Chapter II), etc.

THE EFFECT OF IONISING RADIATION ON THE CELL

Ionising radiation is a corpuscular (e.g. alpha particle) or electromagnetic (e.g. gamma ray, X-ray) radiation which is capable of displacing electrons from atoms or molecules to form ions (which may be positively or negatively charged). These ionised particles have high energy and are destructive to the cell, particularly the nucleus which carries the genetic code and co-ordinates cellular activities. The cellular site of radiation damage was originally considered to be the chromosomes; however, cells which are undergoing rapid division are often more sensitive to radiation *between* divisions, i.e. some process in the manufacture of chromosomal material is sensitive to irradiation rather than the chromosomes themselves. This may possibly be due to impairment of systems by which energy is conserved in the cells, e.g. ionising radiations may uncouple oxidative phosphorylation so that energy is not transferred to produce the energy-rich bonds of ATP but dissipated, hence depriving the cell of its source of energy (this may be of great importance in nuclei where ATP is vital for the polymerisation of bases into the nucleic acids, DNA and RNA, which play a central part in the organisation of the cell). Irradiation also affects the permeability of the membrane of the lysosomes, which contain powerful enzymes, which then leak out into the cell with consequent cellular damage. Whether these are the only ways in which irradiation damages cells is still under consideration.

The effects to man of ionising radiation depend on the dose received, which is traditionally measured in *roentgens* (roentgen is unit of radiation which produces one electrostatic unit per cc. of dry air). However, this is really the exposure dose whereas biological effects are due to the *absorbed dose* of radiation which is the *rad* (one rad means that each gram of matter exposed to radiation absorbs 100 ergs), but this is normally much more difficult to measure and the roentgen (r) is more commonly used as a measure of radiation dosage.

The effects of irradiation in man are summarised below:

Very high dosage (over 5000 r single exposure)—nausea and vomiting followed by death in a day or so usually; if death delayed beyond this then gastro-intestinal damage will soon cause death.

Moderate dosage (800 – 5000 r)—anorexia, nausea and vomiting followed by severe diarrhoea due to gastro-intestinal damage (remember high mitotic rate of gastro-intestinal mucosa—see Chapter VII). Within 2 – 3 weeks marrow aplasia due to radiation damage will cause death (see Chapter V).

Lower dosage (under 800 r single exposure)—less initial nausea but after few weeks damage to haemopoietic tissue will become apparent with reduction in all formed elements in the blood (earliest sign is a fall in the lymphocyte count). This predisposes the person to infection or massive haemorrhage (due to thrombocytopoenia).

The effects of sublethal doses of irradiation over a prolonged period of time are not so clearly defined, although sterility, malignant disease and foetal abnormalities are well documented.

Chapter II

THE ENDOCRINE ORGANS

THE endocrine (ductless) glands secrete substances (hormones) directly into the blood stream. In this section the "conventional" endocrine organs and their physiology and the clinical picture produced by excess or deficiency of their secretion will be studied, but in addition other organs which comply with the above definition (e.g. kidney, pineal) will be mentioned.

THE PITUITARY GLAND

Anterior and posterior lobes.

Embryology—anterior lobe from Rathke's pouch, an outgrowth from the oral cavity and is epithelial; posterior lobe from diverticulum from 3rd ventricle and is nervous tissue.

ANTERIOR LOBE (Adenohypophysis)

The "master" gland of the endocrine system for it produces hormones which affect the other ductless glands.

Secretions— (i) growth (somatotrophic) hormone;
(ii) thyrotrophic hormone (TSH);
(iii) adrenocorticotrophic hormone (ACTH);
(iv) gonadotrophic hormones
follicle-stimulating hormone (FSH):
luteinising hormone (LH), also called interstitial-cell-stimulating hormone (ICSH);
(v) prolactin (lactogenic hormone);
(vi) exophthalmos-producing factor (EPF).

The levels of (i) – (iv) in the plasma can now be measured by means of the radio-immunoassay technique.

Removal: hypophysectomy in animals causes growth arrest, atrophy of thyroid (causing reduced basal metabolic rate, BMR), atrophy of the adrenal cortex (with diminished resistance to stress and infection), atrophy of the gonads.

The clinical picture (panhypopituitarism) may be produced by ischaemic necrosis (e.g. after severe postpartum haemorrhage), a pituitary tumour (craniopharyngioma, chromophobe adenoma), fibrosis or rarer causes (head injury, granulomata like tuberculosis and sarcoidosis). The features are similar to those seen in animals with weakness and lassitude, amenorrhoea and genital atrophy and intolerance to stress (cold, infection).

Disorders of the "target" glands (those on which the pituitary hormones act) may be assessed biochemically:

(*a*) abnormalities of the adrenal cortex—decreased production of glucocorticoids as shown by water load test, sensitivity to hypoglycaemia induced by insulin, reduced urinary excretion of corticosteroid metabolites;

(*b*) abnormalities of the thyroid—decreased level of circulating thyroid hormone, reduced uptake of radioactive iodine. Treatment is by replacement of the secretions (or giving analogues of the hormones) of the target glands.

(i) **Growth hormone.**—A protein from the acidophil cells; necessary for growth for it produces nitrogen retention. Reduced amounts (e.g. panhypopituitarism) lead to growth reduction, and although somatic growth can be changed by the growth hormone, dwarfism is only infrequently caused by primary endocrine abnormalities. In children of small stature due to psychological causes ("deprivation dwarfism") it appears that psychic factors acting via the hypothalamus can depress growth hormone secretion. Little is known about the control of growth hormone secretion, although its release can be stimulated by hypoglycaemia and stress (and there is evidence for the presence of a hypothalamic releasing factor; see Chapter X).

The causes of **dwarfism** are:

Malnutrition (e.g. starvation, specific vitamin deficiencies in scurvy and rickets, malabsorption syndromes such as steatorrhoea);

Chronic illness (e.g. tuberculosis, renal disease, cyanotic congenital heart disease);

Genetic e.g. primordial dwarfism, the "Tom Thumb"; lack of one X chromosome. In African pigmies there is possibly either a resistance to the peripheral action of growth hormone or else they produce a functionally abnormal growth hormone.

Skeletal disorders (e.g. achondroplasia, osteogenesis imperfecta);

Endocrine causes (growth hormone deficiency, thyroxine deficiency).

The presence of excess growth hormone (e.g. due to an acidophil tumour of the pituitary) causes gigantism (when unclosed epiphyses) or acromegaly (in the adult). The clinical picture is typical, but in the acromegalic the excess hormone may cause insulin-resistant diabetes (the diabetogenic effect of growth hormone noted in animals by Houssay).

(ii) **Thyrotrophic stimulating hormone** (TSH).—A protein or polypeptide from basophil cells with a stimulating effect on the thyroid. Its absence (e.g. after hypophysectomy) leads to reduced thyroid activity. Regulation is by nervous influences from the hypothalamus and by a "feed-back" mechanism depending on the blood concentration of thyroid hormone (see Thyroid). In addition there is a TSH "releasing factor" secreted by the hypothalamus (see Chapter X).

(iii) **Adrenocorticotrophic hormone** (ACTH).—A straight chain peptide of 39 amino-acids (molecular weight about 4600) with an effect on the adrenal cortex and controlled both by a blood corticosteroid feed-back mechanism and by a "stress" mechanism via an ACTH-releasing factor (corticotrophin-releasing factor, CRF) produced by the hypothalamus (a polypeptide with molecular weight about 1000) which is secreted into a portal system and carried down by it to the adenohypophysis (see Chapter X). Basophil adenoma leads to excess production of ACTH and hence excess production of adrenal corticosteroids, causing the clinical picture of Cushing's disease (under adrenal cortex).

(iv) **Gonadotrophic hormones** (FSH: LH or ICSH).—FSH causes ripening of ovarian follicles in the female or spermato-genesis in the male. LH is responsible for ovulation and luteinisation, or, as ICSH, for the maintenance of the inter-stitial activity of the testes (and secretion of androgen).

The hypothalamus maintains and regulates the secretion of gonadotrophins probably by producing "releasing factors" which are carried by a portal system from the hypothalamus to the pituitary gland (see Chapter X) (hypothalamic lesions, e.g. pinealoma in boys, can cause sexual precocity and early true puberty, i.e. those "boys" are fertile). Relation to the menstrual cycle is not considered here, but cyclical change in the blood levels of the gonadotrophic hormones is responsible for the regulation of menstruation.

(v) **Prolactin.**—Hypophysectomy (or ischaemic necrosis of

pituitary) prevents the onset of lactation (e.g. Simmond's disease).

(vi) **Exophthalmos-producing hormone.**—Elevated blood level in patients with exophthalmos in thyroid disease, and distinct from changes in the TSH level.

POSTERIOR LOBE (Neurohypophysis)

Together with various nuclei of the hypothalamus really forms one functional unit, the supra-optico-hypophyseal tract. Two hormones are stored in the posterior pituitary:

Oxytocin.—Causes contraction of the uterus; role in physiology unclear but used to stimulate uterus in obstetrical practice (support labour, prevent postpartum haemorrhage); causes ejection of milk from lactating breast.

Antidiuretic hormone (ADH).—Produced in hypothalamus, moves down axons of certain hypophyseal neurones, stored in posterior pituitary and its release is controlled by impulses from the cerebral cortex (fear causes increased ADH release) and from osmoreceptors in the hypothalamus (these osmoreceptors monitor and thereby control the osmotic pressure of the blood; reduced osmotic pressure of the blood, as after drinking water, leads to reduced ADH release and hence a diuresis).

Diabetes insipidus is the clinical syndrome where failure of renal water reabsorption occurs due to an ineffective circulating level of ADH caused by destruction of the posterior pituitary for idiopathic causes or due to infection, trauma, tumours, infiltrations (e.g. sarcoidosis, xanthomatosis as in Hand-Schuller-Christian syndrome) or resistance of the renal tubular cells to the liberated ADH (see Chapter IX).

THE THYROID GLAND

Embryology—median outgrowth from ventral wall of primitive pharynx.

Physiology and biochemistry—profuse blood supply; nerve supply probably has no effect on secretion. The mechanism of production of the iodine-containing hormones, tetra-iodothyronine (thyroxine) and triiodothyronine is given in the figure on the following page.

The major part of plasma thyroxine is bound to the glycoprotein TBP (which is closely related to the protein-bound

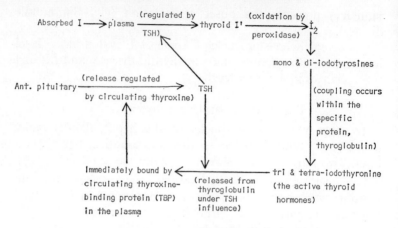

iodine or PBI; an increase in TBP which may occur in normal pregnancy leads to a high PBI but this does not signify thyrotoxicosis; neither does the low PBI in nephrosis, due to urinary loss of TBP, signify hypothyroidism). There are a number of genetically determined defects (all autosomal recessives) of hormonal synthesis producing goitrous cretinism.

Release of preformed thyroid hormone from thyroglobulin is regulated by TSH which in turn is regulated by a "feedback" mechanism, depending on the blood level of thyroxine (see flow diagram above).

The thyroid hormone acts by "uncoupling" the processes whereby oxidative processes in metabolism produce high-energy phosphate bonds (e.g. adenosine triphosphate, ATP) (see Chapter I). When circulating thyroid hormone is present in excess, some of the energy produced by metabolism is lost as heat instead of being used to produce ATP (oxidative metabolic processes are increased to counteract the lack of ATP leading to the increased metabolism seen in thyrotoxicosis).

Experimental thyroidectomy → reduced basal metabolic rate (BMR);

prevents growth (physical and mental) and sexual development in young animals;

reversed by adequate doses of thyroid extract or triiodothyronine.

Hypothyroid States

Cretin.—Deficiency of thyroid hormone in infancy causing a mentally defective dwarf, a cretin, of characteristic appearance. This may be endemic (goitrous child of goitrous mother) due to iodine deficiency in diet, or sporadic (anatomical thyroid defect or autosomal recessive biochemical defect in enzyme formation of which there are at least five types).

Myxoedema.—Adult deficiency of thyroid hormone; reduced mental and physical activity with changes in facial appearance due to thyroid atrophy (spontaneous or following radioactive iodine), thyroid removal (surgery) or as an end stage of an auto-immune process. Thyroid deficiency states can be treated satisfactorily with oral 1-thyroxine.

Goitre.—Major cause of simple goitre (which is a visible or palpable thyroid enlargement) is iodine deficiency, although ingestion of goitrogens (e.g. turnips, swedes), drug therapy (e.g. *p*-aminosalicyclic acid, PAS) or a genetic predisposition account for some. Goitres may have:

> *normal hormone synthesis* being due to iodine lack, growths, thyroiditis;
> *abnormal hormone synthesis* with either hypo- or hyper-function of the thyroid.

A local swelling or solitary nodule of the thyroid is often malignant.

Hyperthyroid States

Thyrotoxicosis (or hyperthyroidism) is a derangement of thyroid function with a failure of homeostasis. The secretion of TSH is diminished together with elevated blood thyroxine levels. In a large number of patients there is evidence for the presence of an abnormal thyroid stimulator ("long acting thyroid stimulator, LATS, which is distinct from TSH and chemically a 7S gamma globulin; its site of production is not yet known). There is some evidence for the presence of an exophthalmos-producing factor (EPF) present at times which is secreted by the pituitary and this may be the prime cause of the exophthalmos (this accounts for the improvement in the exophthalmos seen sometimes following hypophysectomy). A summary of the clinical features of abnormal thyroid states is given on the next page.

BLOOD THYROXINE LEVELS

Effect on	Decreased	Increased
BMR	Reduced BMR (increased weight, cold skin, even hypothermia)	Increased BMR (weight loss, hot skin)
Heart	Bradycardia	Tachycardia
	Abnormal E.C.G. in about 80 per cent	Atrial fibrillation particularly in the elderly
Muscles	Slow relaxation of the ankle jerk	Sometimes weakness of proximal muscles of limb girdle (Thyrotoxic myopathy— see Chapter XI)
Central nervous system	Forgetful, torpid, myxoedema coma	Increased reflexes, fine tremor, labile emotions
Autonomic nervous system	Constipation, dry skin	Diarrhoea, sweating
Childhood	Cretin	
Eyes		Exophthalmos

Treatment of Thyrotoxicosis

(*a*) Drugs e.g. mercazoles (carbimazole) prevent incorporation of iodide into organic radicals (probably by peroxidase inhibition).

(*b*) Surgical removal of part of the thyroid (subtotal thyroidectomy).

(*c*) ^{131}I therapy (radioactive iodine) with destruction of part of the gland by ionising radiation (see Chapter I).

Tests of Thyroid Function

Hormone level in blood (e.g. direct measurement as PBI; butanol extractable iodine, BEI, is an estimate of only thyroxine iodine; indirect measurement by the uptake of radioactive triiodothyronine by red cells or resin).

The kinetics of iodine metabolism (^{131}I or ^{127}I uptake by gland, or the urinary excretion of these isotopes).

Peripheral effects of hormone (e.g. serum cholesterol, BMR,

ankle jerk where there is a delay in relaxation of the ankle jerk in many hypothyroid patients).

Thyrocalcitonin.—A polypeptide hormone produced by the thyroid gland which lowers plasma calcium; it is thought to act by inhibition of bone resorption but it is uncertain whether it plays a part in the physiological homeostasis of calcium. (Its secretion may be increased by a rise in serum calcium concentration although not satisfactorily assessed yet).

PARATHYROID GLANDS

There are now two hormones which directly influence plasma calcium levels:

(a) *Parathyroid hormone*—raises plasma calcium; a polypeptide; origin parathyroid glands which are outgrowths of 3rd and 4th pharyngeal pouches; comes from the chief cells.

(b) *Thyrocalcitonin* (or calcitonin)—reduces plasma calcium; origin ultimobranchial tissue represented in the human by the parafollicular or C cells in the thyroid (although exists as separate glands in some species).

Physiology—plasma calcium is present in three forms—65 per cent ionized, small fraction complexed and diffusible, rest non-diffusible and bound to protein (mainly albumin). Parathyroidectomy in dog causes a fall in plasma calcium, rise in inorganic phosphate, muscle twitching followed by tonic or clonic muscular contractions; the syndrome is known as *tetany*. In man this is characterised by painful limb paraesthesiae followed by involuntary spasm of muscles (positive Trousseau and Chvostek's signs).

Action of hormone—to maintain constancy of plasma ionised calcium; sites of action:

(a) bone—transfers calcium from bone crystals to extracellular fluid;

(b) kidney—reduces tubular reabsorption of phosphorus and increases tubular reabsorption of calcium;

(c) intestine—promotes absorption of calcium.

An increase in serum calcium reduces parathyroid hormone secretion and increases thyrocalcitonin secretion.

Clinical

Hypofunction.—Causes of *tetany* may justifiably be considered here although there are other reasons for tetany than hypoparathyroidism:

(i) hypoparathyroidism, either post-operative (accidental removal) or spontaneous, or where the body is resistant to the action of the hormone (pseudo-hypoparathyroidism);

(ii) rickets and osteomalacia due to vitamin D deficiency or steatorrhoea;

(iii) metabolic alkalosis (e.g. persistent vomiting)

(iv) respiratory alkalosis (e.g. hysterical overbreathing)

⎫ reduction in level of ionised plasma Ca. ⎬

Immediate therapy for tetany is intravenous calcium gluconate; long term therapy is aimed at increasing the absorption of calcium by the intestine using large doses of oral calcium plus vitamin D or dihydrotachysterol, ATIO; or treat the causal disorder.

Hyperfunction.—Usually due to parathyroid adenoma, which causes high plasma calcium (11·0 mg. per cent or above), low plasma phosphorus, increased plasma alkaline phosphatase (only if the bone form of the disease is present) and often increased urinary calcium excretion. Parathyroid hyperfunction presents with renal disorders (calculi, often bilateral, nephrocalcinosis, or renal failure), bone pain, toxic symptoms of hypercalcaemia (reduced appetite, vomiting, thirst, polyuria) and there may be bone rarefraction (especially subperiostial resorption) and cysts.

There are a number of other causes of raised plasma Ca:

(i) malignant disease with bony metastases (e.g. untreated carcinoma of the breast), and rarely without bony metastases (e.g. carcinoma of bronchus which can secrete a parathormone-like substance);

(ii) reticulosis and multiple myelomatosis;

(iii) immobilisation (e.g. poliomyelitis, fractures);

(iv) sarcoidosis (probably produces vitamin D sensitivity) and vitamin D intoxication.

Calcium and Phosphorus Metabolism

Ninety-nine per cent calcium is in bones and teeth while the remainder has various roles (e.g. in blood coagulation, neuro-muscular function, milk production, etc.). It is absorbed from the food (especially diary products) in the upper small intestine under the influence of vitamin D (present in food or produced by the action of ultraviolet light on 7-dehydrocholesterol in the skin); excess intestinal fats reduce calcium absorption (e.g. steatorrhoea, see Chapter VII). Vitamin D is essential for calcium absorption in man but it lowers the renal reabsorption of calcium.

Osteomalacia.—A normal quantity of poorly mineralised bone due to:

   (i) Hypophosphatasia—a recessive disorder with deficiency of alkaline phosphatase in tissues and serum which interferes with the calcification of osteoid tissue.

  (ii) Vitamin D deficiency—reduced dietary intake (with added lack of sunlight) or reduced absorption of vitamin D (steatorrhoea).

 (iii) Renal tubular dysfunction either congenital or acquired (usually a low serum phosphate due to reduced renal tubular reabsorption of phosphate); usually a genetically determined primary defect of the renal tubule but it may be an acquired tubular defect as in galactosaemia and Wilson's disease.

 (iv) Azotaemic renal osteodystrophy may have an element of osteomalacia but this is usually predominantly due to hyperparathyroidism. Bone lesions associated with abnormalities of tubular function occur in three main groups of disorders—renal phosphaturic rickets, renal tubular acidosis, Lignac-Fanconi syndrome.

There is an important relationship between plasma ionised calcium and phosphate such that when one is increased the other tends to fall, which accounts for the importance of lesions of phosphate metabolism in disorders of calcium utilisation. Bone mineralisation does not appear to take place satisfactorily unless the product of calcium and phosphorus is fairly high (usually over 25, but above 60 there is danger of metastatic calcification).

Osteoporosis.—A reduction in the amount of qualitatively normal bone tissue (per unit volume of anatomical bone) resulting in a reduction of the skeletal mass. There are six main causes:

(i) senile or post-menopausal (may be due to reduced secretion of anabolic sex hormones or related to calcium intake but there is really no settled aetiology as yet);

(ii) in young people, e.g. osteogenesis imperfecta, ovarian agenesis (both genetically determined); co-existence with osteomalacia in the intestinal malabsorption syndromes;

(iii) complicating metabolic disorders, e.g. Cushing's syndrome, thyrotoxicosis, acromegaly (the latter is accompanied by hypercalcuria with normal plasma calcium);

(iv) localised, e.g. rheumatoid arthritis, immobilisation in plaster;

(v) reticulosis and neoplasia of the bone marrow;

(vi) idiopathic, either infantile (self-limiting, tendency towards recovery) or adult (with tendency to progression).

THE ADRENAL GLANDS

Two parts, the outer cortex and inner medulla, with different origins and functions.

Embryology—adrenal cortex from urogenital ridge;
adrenal medulla from neural crest.

ADRENAL CORTEX

Anatomy—outer zona glomerulosa (source of aldosterone), middle zona fasciculata and inner zona reticularis. No nerve supply but high concentration of cholesterol in cells (which is required for the synthesis of adrenal steriods).

Physiology

(a) Bilateral adrenalectomy (dogs) causes loss of appetite, weight loss, vomiting, diarrhoea, weakness, prostration, low blood sugar and urinary sodium loss, and finally death.

(b) Bilateral adrenalectomy (dogs) + high salt diet—healthy but unable to resist stress.

Clinical

(a) Above is equivalent to acute adrenal failure in man (e.g. due to meningococcal septicaemia);

(b) above is equivalent to chronic adrenal failure (Addison's disease, e.g. from tuberculosis, autoimmune disease); characterised by asthenia, anorexia and weight loss, hypotension, sensitivity to stresses (such as cold and infections) and skin pigmentation.

Hormones.—All steroids have a common molecular structure of 17 carbon atoms known as the cyclopentenophenanthrene nucleus and there are only three major groups based on physiological action:

  (i) glucocorticoids;
  (ii) mineralocorticoids;
  (iii) androgenic steroids.

(i) *Glucocorticoids*—(contain 21 carbon atoms and called C_{21} steroids); main hormones are hydrocortisone and corticosterone (in man the ratio is about $8:1$); their secretion is regulated by pituitary ACTH (the diurnal variation in hydrocortisone secretion in man, with maximum level between 4 and 8 a.m., is due to a diurnal rhythm in the secretion of ACTH). Hydrocortisone is normally carried reversibly bound to a specific α-globulin and metabolised by the liver. It affects carbohydrate metabolism and causes deposition of glycogen in the liver; it causes the breakdown of tissue proteins with the production of glucose (gluconeogenesis); the glucocorticoids are also involved in protection of the body against stress. Both hydrocortisone (cortisol) and aldosterone are concerned with the internal distribution of water and electrolytes between extracellular and intracellular compartments.

Deficiency (*Addison's disease*)—low blood sugar, low blood pressure (presumably due to reduced aldosterone secretion mainly), unable to resist stress, pigmentation (due to excess production of ACTH and/or a melanophore-stimulating hormone in an attempt to increase adrenal cortical secretion but also stimulating skin melanophores).

Excess secretion (*Cushing's syndrome*)—either primary excess ACTH production from pituitary basophil adenomata (rarely ACTH-like material from oat-cell carcinoma of bronchus) or a primary tumour of the adrenal cortex. Protein catabolism is the key to the clinical picture, and there is muscle wasting, weakness, osteoporosis, gluconeogenesis (and hence diabetes), and hypertension, characteristic body habitus and facies (latter due to androgenic steroids partly) with increased urinary excretion of 17-hydroxycorticoids (hydrocortisone is a 17-hydroxycorticoid which means a hydroxyl group on No. 17 carbon atom of the steroid nucleus drawn here).

STEROID   NUCLEUS

(ii) *Mineralocorticoids*—(C_{21} steroids) aldosterone (named because of aldehyde group on No. 18 carbon atom); active in control of water and mineral metabolism by regulating the balance of sodium in the body (acts mainly on the distal tubules of the kidney to promote renal tubular reabsorption of Na^+ in exchange for K^+). Its secretion is regulated by the following mechanisms:

ACTH secretion by pituitary;

renin-angiotensin system of kidney;

probably by intracellular sodium content of cells of zona glomerulosa.

Deficiency causes reduced tubular reabsorption of Na^+ with consequent Na^+ loss from body leading to dehydration on account of concomitant water loss, and reduced blood pressure, e.g. uncontrolled Addison's disease.

Excess (e.g. primary hyperaldosteronism or Conn's syndrome); plasma sodium may increase but oedema is uncommon (unexplained), hypertension, but really potassium loss dominates (causing muscle weakness). Hyperaldosteronism is seen secondary to malignant hypertension (because of excess renin release from destruction of kidney tissue), congestive heart failure (excess renin release and reduced inactivation of aldosterone by the liver) and cirrhosis of liver (partly due to reduced inactivation of aldosterone).

(iii) *Androgenic steroids*—C_{19} steroids and no side chain on No. 17 carbon atom; main one is dehydro-epiandrosterone, but these androgens are not so potent as their testicular counterparts. Their main effect is protein anabolism and the production of secondary male sexual characteristics (accounting for facial hair in Cushing's syndrome).

Physiology—flow diagram below shows how adrenal corticosteroids are produced and many enzymes in the adrenal cortical cells are required for these steps:

$$\text{cholesterol} \xrightarrow{} \text{pregnenolone} \xrightarrow{} \text{progesterone} \xrightarrow{} \begin{array}{l}\text{hydrocortisone}\\\text{corticosterone}\\\text{aldosterone}\end{array}$$

$$\downarrow C_{19} \qquad C_{21}$$

androgenic steroids

The conjugated metabolites of the adrenal androgens are 17-oxosteroids.

Clinical—enzyme deficiencies after the progesterone stage cause increased ACTH secretion (because of a low blood level of hydrocortisone activating the production of ACTH by the pituitary), bilateral adrenocortical hyperplasia and hence excess production of C_{19} androgenic steroids. Excess androgenic steroid production will produce genital deformity in a female child, *pseudohermaphroditism* (depending on phase of development when the excess androgen secretion starts; there is also the possibility of insufficient production of other adrenal steroids), and *sexual precocity* in male; there may be severe adrenal insufficiency if the metabolic block is almost complete. A milder form is seen in girls at puberty due to excess androgens, but not Addisonian features (the *adrenogenital syndrome*) which can be suppressed by exogenous steroids.

Adrenal Cortical Function Tests

Tests of basal secretory activity:

(i) plasma hydrocortisone level;

(ii) hydrocortisone secretion rate;

(iii) free or conjugated corticosteroids in the urine; metabolites of hydrocortisone are mainly conjugated with glucuronic acid and estimated as 17-oxogenic steroids (used to be called 17-ketogenic steroids).

Stimulation tests:

(i) of adrenal hormone production, e.g. using ACTH which indicates the degree of adrenal hypofunction present but does not give information about the ability of the pituitary to produce and secrete ACTH;

(ii) of pituitary ACTH release, e.g. the "stress" mechanism (using hypoglycaemia), e.g. the feedback mechanism using metyrapone (which is a specific 11β-hydroxylase inhibitor acting on the adrenal cortex which produces a fall in plasma hydrocortisone level and will cause a release of ACTH to give a rise in urinary 17-oxogenic steroids in normal subjects), e.g. using vasopressin (either similar to corticotrophin-releasing factor or actually causes CRF to be released) which will produce a rise in plasma hydrocortisone level.

Suppression tests which are used to evaluate adrenal hyperfunction e.g. using dexamethasone.

Adrenal Medulla

It forms part of the sympathetic nervous system, being supplied by *preganglionic* sympathetic fibres; secretes adrenaline and noradrenaline (latter really adrenaline without methyl group; they have similar actions except adrenaline has a greater metabolic effect, e.g. on blood sugar and many tissues, causes vasodilation of muscle blood vessels and therefore is a much less powerful pressor agent than noradrenaline. Both have similar stimulating effects on the heart to increase stroke volume, but adrenaline increases heart rate without increasing blood pressure, whereas noradrenaline does not cause tachycardia due to reflex vagal inhibition of the heart rate following the increase in blood pressure consequent on the vasoconstriction of arterioles).

Clinical—tumour of chromaffin (i.e. chromium-staining) cells of medulla (phaeochromocytoma) causing paroxysmal or sustained hypertension and possibly with other features such as sweating, transient glycosuria, anxiety (due mainly to the greater metabolic action of adrenaline). The symptoms seen are due to varying increases in adrenaline and noradrenaline secretion which can be detected in blood or urine (or else by estimating a breakdown product, vanilmandelic acid, VMA, which is measured in the urine). Adrenergic antagonists (e.g. the α-blocking agent phentolamine) can be used to block the catecholamine effect and produce a significant fall in blood pressure when a phaeochromocytoma is present.

In benign hypertension, blocking the action of noradrenaline at postganglionic sympathetic nerve endings (e.g. with methyldopa) can relax arterioles, reduce total peripheral resistance and hence lead to a fall in blood pressure (see Chapter X).

KIDNEY

The kidney secretes two humoral materials at least:

   (i) renin—an enzyme (protein);
  (ii) erythropoietin—a glycoprotein.

   (i) **Renin.**—Secreted by the juxtaglomerular cells (J-G cells) in the wall of the afferent arterioles of the renal glomerulus in response to reduced blood flow and/or reduced pulse pressure (possibly reduced perfusion pressure); it has an enzymic action on a plasma substrate with the eventual formation of the octapeptide, angiotensin II, which, besides being a very potent pressor agent, is a stimulus for the release of aldosterone from the adrenal cortex. More recently renin release has been noted to occur in response to changes in the composition of fluid in the kidney tubule (particularly Na^+), possibly acting via the macula densa (the formation of angiotensin from renin may then adjust the filtration rate through the glomerulus so as to adjust the renal tubular sodium load).

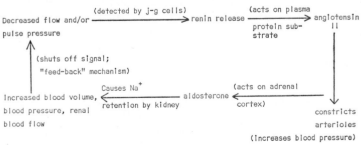

Clinical—important in malignant hypertension where renin level in blood is raised; also causes secondary hyperaldosteronism and may be important in the hypertension of renal artery stenosis; it also has some ill-defined role in the reaction of the body to "shock".

The kidney also has a hypotensive action (? humoral) for removal of *both* kidneys can produce hypertension (renoprival hypertension) and also in renal transplanatation there is often an immediate fall in previously high blood pressure in the recipient when the kidney is implanted.

(ii) **Erythropoietin.**

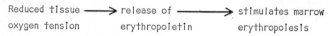

Reduced tissue ⟶ release of ⟶ stimulates marrow
oxygen tension   erythropoietin   erythropoiesis

Clinical—polycythaemia may occur in certain renal tumours (e.g. hypernephroma) and there is an increased blood level of erythropoietin in many anaemias, although that due to renal disease is not one of them.

THYMUS

To restore immune mechanisms after thymectomy in the newborn animal it is necessary to inject or graft lymphoid or thymus tissue, and in the case of the latter this appears to be mediated by a humoral factor not yet elucidated.

PINEAL

Melatonin is a mammalian humoral material released from the pineal and it has an effect on the oestrus cycle by slowing it down.

Clinical—pineal tumours in boys may lead to true (i.e. fertile) precocious puberty, but these tumours are now considered not to be true pineal tumours but rather come from surrounding structures, press on the pineal and reduce the amount of melatonin, or some similar antigonadal hormone, secreted and hence cause precocious puberty.

GASTRIN, SECRETIN, PANCREOZYMIN, CHOLECYSTOKININ

These are gastro-intestinal tract hormones (see Chapter VII).

PANCREAS

The secretions of the pancreas are:

Exocrine.—Into the duodenum and concerned with digestion of food (see Chapter VII).

Endocrine.—At least two hormones are secreted into the blood by the pancreas:

(*a*) *insulin*—composed of two peptide chains of amino-acids; molecular weight only 12,000; injection produces a fall in blood glucose by promoting glucose utilisation by the cells of the body (primarily stimulates transfer of glucose across the cell wall);

(*b*) *glucagon*—produced by α-cells of islets of Langerhans (insulin from the β-cells) and produces hyperglycaemia by promoting hepatic glycogenolysis;

(*c*) *gastrin* can be produced in excessive amounts by non-insulin secreting islet cell pancreatic tumours (the Zollinger-Ellison syndrome—see Chapter VII.)

Regulation of blood glucose—i.e the balance between the entry of glucose into the blood and its metabolism by the body cells. Glucose enters the blood from:

the small intestine (digestion of dietary carbohydrates);

the liver (by breakdown of glycogen—*glycogenolysis*, and formation from amino-acids—*gluconeogenesis*).

The blood glucose level is controlled by insulin which may circulate in free form or bound to protein, and insulin is destroyed by an enzyme, insulinase, in the liver and kidneys. Several hormones act in response to a drop in blood glucose level (adrenaline, glucagon, glucocorticoids, growth hormone) but only insulin is known to respond to a rise. These hormonal regulators combine to ensure that blood glucose rarely falls below critical levels.

Diabetes mellitus is a syndrome due to an absolute or relative deficiency of insulin available for use by the cells of the body and this may be due to reduced pancreatic secretion or due to influence of insulin-antagonists in the plasma. As in many diabetics a reduced plasma insulin cannot be detected, the primary abnormality in diabetes mellitus may well be an excessive level of insulin antagonists in the blood.

Diabetes mellitus may manifest itself as a severe form

associated with ketosis ("juvenile" type) (accumulation of keto acids and acetone in the blood) in which insulin is essential for life, or a milder form ("maturity onset" type) associated with obesity and often controlled by dietary carbohydrate restriction and consquent weight reduction. The clinical and biochemical features of diabetes depend on hyperglycaemia, but the cause of the degenerative complications seen with long-standing diabetes is unclear (these include cataracts, retinopathy, neuropathy, nephropathy and atherosclerosis). The formation of excess ketone bodies in the patient in untreated severe diabetes is due to the biochemical coupling between fatty acid metabolism and glucose metabolism (see Chapter I) which supply energy for cell metabolism. When glucose metabolism is impaired in diabetes mellitus the energy requirements of the body cells are met by an increase in fat oxidation with the formation of excessive amounts of ketone bodies (β-hydroxybutyric acid, acetoacetic acid and acetone).

TESTIS

The main androgen (or male sex hormone) is testosterone which is a C19 steroid (no side chain at 17th carbon atom of the nucleus). The biosynthetic pathway is:

Cholesterol—Progesterone—17-OH progesterone—
testosterone.

It causes development of the secondary male sexual characteristics and has a protein anabolic effect. It is synthesised from cholesterol in the Leydig cells of the testis under the control of the hypophysis (the *interstitial cell-stimulating hormone*, ICSH) and there is a negative feedback such that elevated blood androgen levels inhibit ICSH release (this feedback is really at the level of the hypothalamus).

Hypogonadism (testicular failure) may result from:

(*a*) Primary disorder of the testis, e.g. disease (mumps), trauma, infiltration (haemachromatosis), chromosomal anomaly (XXY of Klinefelter's syndrome), idiopathic.

(*b*) Pituitary gonadotrophin insufficiency, e.g. secondary to chronic illness, or organic or functional lesion of pituitary.

Certain testicular tumours occur which secrete hormones in excessive amounts:

(i) Teratoma—chorionic gonadotrophin.
(ii) Leydig cell tumour—androgens (causes precocious puberty).
(iii) Sertoli cell tumour—oestrogens (causes feminisation: testis normally produces oestrogens whose function is unknown).

OVARY

The cells of the ovarian follicle produce oestrogens and progesterone, and the number of follicles developing simultaneously can be increased by injecting human pituitary gonadotrophin preparation (and hence cause multiple pregnancies).

Oestrogens cause female secondary sexual characteristics and duct growth of the breast; they are responsible for oestrous behaviour in animals, produce cyclical changes in the endometrium, cervix and vagina in the human and also may produce Na^+ (and water) retention (leading to premenstrual tension syndrome).

Oestradiol is synthesised from progesterone under the control of the *follicle-stimulating hormone* (FSH) from the anterior pituitary (promotes maturation of follicular cells as well as oestrogen secretion).

Progesterone is a C_{21} steroid secreted by the corpus luteum (and placenta) and this is regulated by the *luteotrophic hormone*

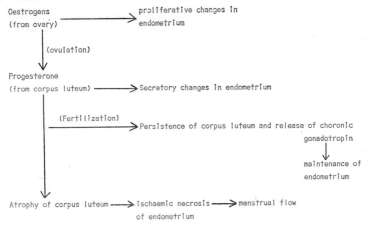

(LH) from the anterior pituitary. It stimulates secretory changes in the endometrium and development of lobules and alveoli of the breast. Synthetic progestational agents are used orally to block LH secretion and prevent ovulation (i.e. act as contraceptives).

The cyclic production of oestrogens and progesterone are responsible for the *menstrual cycle* in humans: (see page 29)

The failure of the ovaries to produce their hormones (in spite of high blood gonadotrophin levels) is responsible for the menopause after which the menstrual cycle ceases. Menstrual disorders will not be discussed here, but there are certain disorders of ovarian function of interest:

(i) androgen-producing ovarian tumour (arrhenoblastoma) will cause virilism;

(ii) Stein-Leventhal syndrome—defect in oestrogen synthesis with increased androgen production which causes virilism and sterility;

(iii) failure of ovarian development due to primary gonadal defect as in Turner's syndrome where there is only one X chromosome (XO);

(iv) failure of ovaries at the menopause ("just worn out").

PLACENTA

In pregnancy large amounts of *chorionic gonadotrophin* are produced by the placenta; this differs from pituitary gonadotrophic extracts in that it does not have the effects on stimulating ovarian growth but has mainly a luteinizing action. The active principle is probably a high molecular weight glycoprotein (M. Wt. c. 100,000), but the mechanism controlling its release is unknown. Human chorionic gonadotrophin (HCG) excretion in the urine in pregnancy is detected by a variety of pregnancy diagnosis tests (e.g. Aschheim-Zondek test using immature mice, Friedman test using rabbits, injection into Xenopus toad in Hogben test, and now a latex precipitation test; in the latter, rabbit antiserum against HCG is prepared and incubated with urine and then latex particles coated with HCG are added and if they remain in suspension the test is positive).

There are other hormones from the placenta, one called *placental lactogen* with growth hormone-like biochemical action (in relatively high concentrations in plasma in pregnancy) and another called *chorionic thyrotrophic hormone.*

Chapter III

CARDIOVASCULAR SYSTEM

CARDIAC MUSCLE

DUE to the unequal distribution of ions across the cell membrane, the interior of a cardiac muscle fibre is 80 – 90 millivolts negative to an indifferent electrode; depolarisation (with some reversal of polarity) occurs following stimulation, then repolarisation takes place to restore the original state of polarity (see Chapter X). The duration of this action potential is related to the heart rate (faster the rate, the shorter the duration). The action potential of cardiac muscle differs from that of nerve or skeletal muscle in its greater duration and in the great variability of duration with rate. There is a close temporal relationship between mechanical and electrical activity with contraction commencing a few milliseconds after depolarisation (and usually the contraction time is approximately equal to the duration of the action potential).

Cardiac muscle has the general properties and characteristics of skeletal muscle (see Chapter XI) but does have an inherent rhythmicity of its own and will beat when completely denervated. The heart is composed of individual muscle cells but these function as if they were all one cell, i.e. the heart behaves as a functional syncytium. The nerves to the heart alter this rhythmic contraction in relation to the need of the body. Cardiac muscle has this inherent rhythmicity which is normally altered by certain pacemaker areas (here specialised cells depolarise more frequently than does cardiac muscle and hence dominate the frequency of depolarisation of the myocardium, e.g. sino-atrial or SA node, and atrioventricular, AV node). Contraction of cardiac muscle is followed by an absolute refractory period (in which no stimulus can evoke a contraction) and then a relative refractory period. As the cardiac cell membrane is refractory to further stimulation until repolarisation is well advanced there can be no summation in cardiac muscle. However, if a pair of stimuli are so spaced that the second occurs shortly after the refractory period of the first, it is possible to produce a condition in which only a single mechanical beat results from each pair of depolarisations (*paired pulse stimulation*); this has been used clinically to lengthen the absolute refractory period (for controlled slowing of the heart rate) and also to increase the mechanical power of the beat (in this case electrical depolarisation is equivalent to an extrasystole and the resultant mechanical beat shows postextrasystolic potentiation; this increased beat does not cause any significant change in cardiac output and there is an increased oxygen consumption by the heart so the procedure is probably of no use clinically to improve cardiac performance).

The mechanical characteristics of muscle are dealt with in Chapter XI and cardiac muscle follows the general rule for length-tension relationships (Starling's Law of the Heart is a specific application of this), and its basic cell structure is considered very similar to that of skeletal muscle.

Clinical disorders of cardiac action can be broadly grouped into those:

(i) concerned with changes in the rate, rhythm and conduction in the heart;

(ii) due to changes in the capability of the cardiac muscle to contract.

In the latter group, damage to the muscle may be due to well-known disorders such as atherosclerosis which reduces myocardial blood supply (and hence damages contractile machinery), but there is a group of less well understood disorders affecting the cardiac muscle directly which are collected together under the term cardiomyopathy.

CARDIOMYOPATHIES

These are disorders of cardiac muscle function not due to atherosclerotic, rheumatic, luetic, pulmonary or congenital heart disease, and more easily understood when the title "*primary myocardial disease*" is used (for the myocardium, and sometimes endocardium, are the structures primarily affected by the disorder). There are many known causes (given below) but in many patients the causative factor cannot be defined at present. The heart may be primarily affected (primary) or be affected as part of a generalised disease (secondary).

Primary Cardiomyopathies

(i) infections, e.g. viruses such as Coxsackie B, influenza;

(ii) alcoholic cardiomyopathy in which improvement occurs with abstinence from alcohol;

(iii) endomyocardial fibrosis which is a common cardio-myopathy in East and West Africans in which the normal endocardial lining of the heart is replaced by abnormal fibrous tissue;

(iv) endocardial fibroelastosis occurs in the first year of life and causes progressive heart failure due to a thick white layer of fibrous tissue covering the endocardium;

(v) puerperal cardiomyopathy in which fibrosis and hyalinisa-tion of muscle fibres of the heart occurs with some inflammatory changes; this may not really be specific to the postpartum period but could be of infectious aetiology;

(vi) hypertrophic obstructive cardiomyopathy where there is diffuse muscular hypertrophy of the left ventricular outflow tract in particular of unknown aetiology.

Secondary Cardiomyopathies

A generalised disease affecting other organs as well as the heart:

(i) infections, e.g. virus, protozoa (toxoplasmosis, Chaga's disease);

(ii) infiltrations, e.g. amyloidosis, haemochromatosis;

(iii) endocrine, e.g. thyrotoxicosis;

(iv) damage to blood vessels, especially in the connective tissue disorders, e.g. systemic lupus erythematosis, polyarteritis nodosa, diffuse systemic sclerosis;

(v) neurological, e.g. Friedreich's ataxia;

(vi) sarcoidosis.

PACEMAKERS

The inherent automacity of cardiac muscle can be altered by impulses from the SA or AV nodes which depolarise spontaneously. The difference between the transmembrane potential of a pacemaker cell and a fibre of either atrial or ventricular muscle is that the pacemaker depolarises more frequently than ordinary cardiac muscle and produces an action potential which then depolarises the entire cardiac muscle, leading to contraction of the heart. Although the heart is composed of individual muscle cells these function as if they were all one cell, i.e. the heart behaves as a functional *syncytium*. All cardiac muscle cells are capable of spontaneous depolarisation due to a leakage of Na$^+$ ions across the membrane of the muscle cells (see Chapter X on the properties of excitable membranes), but in the case of pacemaker cells this sodium leak is more rapid so that they depolarise at a higher rate (and hence higher frequency) than does the atrial or ventricular muscle. The sympathetic nerves to the pacemaker cells (or sympathomimetic amines) increase the rate of spontaneous depolarisation (hence

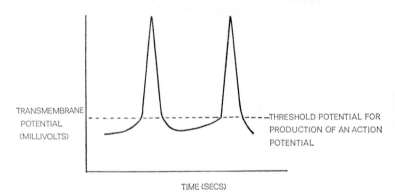

TRANSMEMBRANE POTENTIAL (MILLIVOLTS)

THRESHOLD POTENTIAL FOR PRODUCTION OF AN ACTION POTENTIAL

TIME (SECS)

RHYTHMICAL DISCHARGE OF AN S-A NODAL FIBRE

FIG. 1.

increase heart rate) while the vagi (or acetylcholine) decrease the rate of spontaneous depolarisation (reduce the heart rate). Pacing the heart, normally accomplished via the nerves to the heart (sympathetic and parasympathetic), can be done artificially by the application of a depolarising current directly to the myocardium (e.g. using a catheter inserted into the right ventricle through the external jugular vein, or else by attaching wires to the myocardium externally with the pacemaker being inserted into the anterior abdominal wall; the current required for myocardial pacing is approximately 8 milliamperes at a peak voltage of 8 volts for about 2 milliseconds).

When a spontaneous potential occurs in the SA node it spreads to the atria, then through the AV node into the ventricles, causing all parts of the heart to contract at the rhythmical rate of the SA node which is normally about 70 – 80 beats per minute; if the SA node fails to generate impulses the AV node or part of the Purkinje system will become the pacemaker; also a damaged area of heart muscle in the atria or ventricles can become very irritable, develop a rate of spontaneous depolarisation greater than the SA node and interfere with the normal rhythmicity of the heart (e.g. atrial fibrillation, ventricular tachycardia).

VARIATIONS IN CARDIAC RHYTHM

Changes in heart rate governed by the SA node:

sinus arrhythmia (heart rate increases with inspiration, decreases with expiration);

sinus tachycardia (usually due to increased sympathetic impulses to the heart);

sinus bradycardia (increased parasympathetic tone, i.e. vagal impulses to the heart);

sino-atrial block (partial or complete failure of SA node to generate impulses).

Ectopic beats.—These are premature cardiac contractions induced by the discharge of some ectopic impulse-forming focus anywhere in the heart:

atrial extrasystoles;

nodal extrasystoles;

ventricular extrasystoles.

Tachycardias.—Ectopic beats occur in rapid succession.

(i) Paroxysmal atrial tachycardia (rate 150 – 220/min. and of abrupt onset);

(ii) atrial flutter (rapid atrial pulsation of 180 – 360/min. usually with block by AV node so that ventricles beat at a fraction of this rate, e.g. half, quarter);

(iii) atrial fibrillation (irregular ventricular rate of approximately 150 – 300/min.);

(iv) ventricular tachycardia (regular ventricular rate of approximately 150 – 300/min.);

(v) ventricular fibrillation (irregular ventricular movement without effective contraction).

These tachycardias are of haemodynamic importance as they reduce cardiac output which is most marked with ventricular fibrillation where the cardiac output is zero; ventricular tachycardia has a greater effect on cardiac output than atrial arrhythmias with a similar ventricular rate although atrial fibrillation may reduce cardiac output markedly (removal of effective atrial systole probably reduces cardiac output only 5 – 15 per cent but the rapid ventricular rate with poor ventricular filling may interfere with cardiac output to a much greater extent in atrial fibrillation).

Disorders of conduction where the excitatory impulse may be delayed, interrupted or changed from its usual path during its passage from SA node to the ventricles.

Heart block (conduction at AV node or through the bundle of His is delayed or blocked completely); this may be partial or complete;

bundle-branch block—delayed conduction of the excitatory impulse to either right or left ventricle;

intraventricular block—e.g. peri-infarction block where the sequence of depolarisation in the ventricle is altered without prolongation of QRS interval;

Wolff-Parkinson-White syndrome—the excitatory impulse travels by an anomalous pathway from atrium to ventricle.

ELECTROCARDIOGRAPHY

The movement of charged particles (ions) across the membrane of the myocardial cells produces a flow of electrical current which can be recorded by a galvanometer to produce a graphic record, the electrocardiogram (ECG). The electrical events which produce the ECG are summarised below:

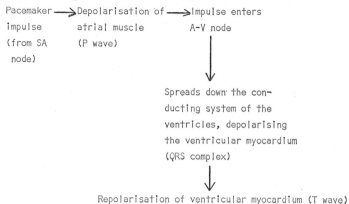

```
Pacemaker ———→ Depolarisation of ———→ Impulse enters
impulse              atrial muscle              A-V node
(from SA            (P wave)
node)
                                                      |
                                                      ↓
                                         Spreads down the con-
                                         ducting system of the
                                         ventricles, depolarising
                                         the ventricular myocardium
                                         (QRS complex)
                                                      |
                                                      ↓
                        Repolarisation of ventricular myocardium (T wave)
```

Interpretation of the standard bipolar leads of the ECG proved empirical until Wilson's introduction of a neutral electrode which is the basis of the "V" leads. The study of electrocardiography will not be discussed further here, being adequately covered in specialised books.

THE CARDIAC CYCLE

Blood delivered by the great veins to the right atrium flows into the right ventricle, being partly forced in by right atrial systole through the tricuspid valve.

Right Atrium and Jugular Venous Pulse

The pressure changes which occur in the right atrium during the cardiac cycle are well displayed in the internal jugular venous pulse while the height of blood in the external jugular vein is more a measure of the mean right atrial pressure. The jugular venous pulse (better seen in internal jugular vein) has the following wave form:

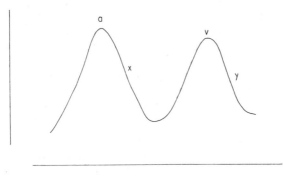

JUGULAR VENOUS PULSE

a is due to the right atrial systole;

x descent—tricuspid valve and atrioventricular septum drawn down by right ventricular systole (c wave which interrupts x descent should be ignored);

v wave—rising right atrial pressure due to temporary obstruction to blood flow by closure of tricuspid valve during right ventricular systole;

y descent—opening of tricuspid valve and blood flows into the right ventricle.

Jugular venous pressure is measured with reference to the sternal angle which is 5 cm. above the centre of the right atrium; with the patient at 45° to the horizontal the top of the column of blood in the external jugular vein (representing the mean venous pressure) is at or below the level of the clavicle in health. The mean right atrial pressure is increased in congestive heart failure, by increased intrathoracic pressure (e.g. straining), raised intrapericardial pressure, obstruction to venous inflow into the heart; the first cause in the most important one.

Abnormalities of the wave form of the jugular venous pulse:

(a) the *a* wave disappears in atrial fibrillation (no atrial systole) and is increased in size when there is resistance to the outflow of blood in atrial systole (e.g. tricuspid stenosis or atresia, increased right ventricular end-diastolic pressure because of severe pulmonary hypertension or pulmonary stenosis). Remember it is presystolic in timing (i.e. occurs prior to the carotid impulse which is due to left ventricular systole). Cannon waves occur when the right atrium contracts against a closed tricupsid valve (e.g. complete heart block);

(b) *x* descent—not clearly seen in atrial fibrillation and diminished in tricuspid incompetence;

(c) *v* waves—very large in tricuspid incompetence;

(d) *y* descent—very rapid (diastolic collapse) in constrictive pericarditis and tricuspid incompetence, whereas it is slow in tricuspid stenosis. Understanding the genesis of the jugular venous pulse is the key to the interpretation of right-sided cardiac lesions.

Right Ventricle and Pulmonary Artery

The right ventricle pumps against the pulmonary circuit, a low resistance vascular tree at a pressure of about 30/10 mm.Hg, and this accounts for the smaller thickness of the right ventricular myocardium compared with that of the left ventricle; with inspiration the right ventricular output increases and there is a slight prolongation in the ejection phase (i.e. prolongation of right ventricular systole during inspiration as more blood flows into the right ventricle which influences the degree of splitting of the second heart sound).

Murmurs are due to turbulent flow through narrowed and/or incompetent valves, the main right-sided murmurs being:

(i) presystolic murmur of tricuspid stenosis (increased by inspiration);

(ii) pansystolic murmur of tricuspid incompetence (increased by inspiration);

(iii) systolic murmur produced by increased flow across the pulmonary valve as in atrial septal defect (ASD);

(iv) turbulence due to idiopathic dilatation of the pulmonary artery can produce a systolic murmur;

(v) pulmonary systolic murmur due to stenosis of infundibulum of the right ventricle or pulmonary valve;

(vi) stenosis above the pulmonary valve as in supravalvular pulmonary stenosis and multiple branch stenosis of the pulmonary artery which both cause ejection type (i.e. diamond shaped) systolic murmurs;

(vii) diastolic murmur of pulmonary incompetence which may be congenital in origin or else functional due to pulmonary hypertension (Graham Steell murmur).

Left Atrium

After leaving the pulmonary circuit blood enters the left atrium, traverses the mitral valve (being aided by left atrial systole) and enters the left ventricle, from which it is expelled via the aortic valve into the aorta. Its distribution from thence depends on the characteristics of the local vascular circuits and these will be considered later.

The pressure changes in the left atrium can be obtained by inserting a catheter directly into this chamber (e.g. from the right atrium via the fossa ovale) or indirectly from an occluded small pulmonary artery ("wedge pressure"). The waves are of similar origin to those in the right atrium and are called a and v waves (a being due to left atrial systole, v occurs during left ventricular systole). Abnormalities in the size or shape of the left atrial pressure trace are:

(i) large a wave due to mitral stenosis which disappears when atrial fibrillation is also present;

(ii) large v wave when mitral regurgitation occurs.

The normal pressures are approximately a mean of 8 mm.Hg, a wave peak 10 mm.Hg, v wave 12 mm.Hg (measured from 5 cm. below sternal angle).

Left Ventricle

In the left ventricle the diastolic pressure is usually below 10 mm.Hg and the systolic pressure is the same as the aortic systolic pressure in the absence of obstruction to left ventricular outflow. When the end-diastolic pressure of the left ventricle increases the muscle fibres are stretched and according to Starling's Law of the Heart (see later) more work can be done by the left ventricular muscle. This is seen when there is heart failure and greater "stretching" of muscle fibres is required to do the ordinary work of the heart due to strain on, or disease of, the myocardium. Murmurs generated on the left side of the heart are:

   (i) mid-diastolic murmur due to blood flow through a narrowed mitral valve (mitral stenosis);

  (ii) apical diastolic murmur due to abnormalities (stenosis or inflammation) of the mitral valve (e.g. Carey Coombs murmur);

 (iii) presystolic murmurs of mitral stenosis due to left atrial systole (absent in atrial fibrillation);

 (iv) early diastolic murmur of aortic incompetence;

  (v) presystolic murmur in aortic incompetence (Austin Flint murmur) due to vibration of the anterior or aortic leaflet of the mitral valve;

 (vi) pansystolic murmur of mitral incompetence due to rheumatic heart disease or papillary muscle dysfunction (the murmur may be late in systole or even represented by multiple systolic clicks);

(vii) systolic murmur of left ventricular outflow obstruction from subvalvular (infundibular) obstruction by a band or hypertrophied muscle (latter is called obstructive cardiomyopathy), aortic valve stenosis or supravalvular aortic stenosis.

Peripheral artery.—The pulsation following the ejection of blood from the left ventricle is transmitted through the arteries and felt as the pulse wave which may be studied as regards frequency, regularity and form.

Frequency and regularity:	increased and regular in sinus tachycardia, atrial flutter with AV block, ventricular tachycardia;
	decreased and regular in sinus bradycardia, complete heart block;
	irregular in atrial fibrillation, frequent extrasystoles (either ventricular or supraventricular in origin), sinus arrhythmia.

Form: absent when no blood flow as in cardiac arrest or
           blocked artery (reduced in partial obstruction to
           artery as in coarctation of the aorta);
           small amplitude due to low cardiac output as in shock,
           severe aortic or mitral stenosis;
           increased amplitude, i.e. increased pulse pressure, as in
           aortic incompetence, excitement, thyrotoxicosis;
           slow upstroke in aortic stenosis (heart has difficulty
           ejecting blood from the left ventricle);
           bisferiens in combined aortic stenosis and incompetence;
           pulsus alternans (alternate large and small pulse waves)
           in left ventricular failure);
           pulsus paradoxicus in which the pulse may disappear on
           inspiration (normally quickens), e.g. pericardial
           effusion;
           pulsus bigeminus due to alternate ventricular ectopic
           beats.

APEX CARDIOGRAPHY

The movements of the left ventricle can be graphically
recorded as the apex cardiogram (ACG) which is shown in
diagram form below:

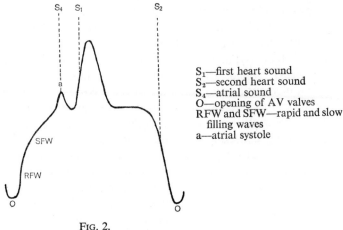

S₁—first heart sound
S₂—second heart sound
S₄—atrial sound
O—opening of AV valves
RFW and SFW—rapid and slow
   filling waves
a—atrial systole

FIG. 2.

The apex cardiogram is of great assistance in the identification
of the diastolic events of the cardiac cycle. The relationship

between heart sounds and movements of the left ventricle (as recorded by the ACG) are seen above.

Murmurs produced by abnormal connections between the heart chambers or great vessels:

(a) atrial septal defect—no murmur due to blood flow from left to right atrium (murmur due to excessive flow of blood through the pulmonary valve in ASD);

(b) ventricular septal defect—pansystolic murmur as blood flows from high pressure left ventricle to low pressure right ventricle in systole;

(c) aorto-pulmonary connection, either aorto-pulmonary window or patent ductus arteriosus, when blood flows in systole and diastole from high pressure aorta to lower pressure pulmonary artery ("continuous or machinery murmur").

These murmurs change their characteristics when the pulmonary artery (and right ventricular) pressure increases due to an increase in pulmonary vascular resistance.

Cardiac Cycle and Origin of Heart Sounds

First heart sound (S_1)—due to mitral and tricuspid valve closure (mitral before tricuspid) and the intensity is increased when the valve leaflets are wide open immediately before the ventricle contracts (short P-R interval, hyperkinetic circulatory states, mitral stenosis); may be a split first heart sound in health.

Second heart sound (S_2)—aortic and pulmonary valve closure (first element aortic) and a lag of the second component (P2 or pulmonary valve closure) occurs with inspiration due to prolongation of right ventricular systole from increased right ventricular filling consequent on the increased negative intra-thoracic pressure at inspiration. Delay in pulmonary valve closure (increased splitting) occurs in right bundle branch block (delayed activation of the right ventricle), pulmonary stenosis and atrial septal defect (increased right ventricular work or flow with consequent increased duration of right ventricular systole). In aortic stenosis and with left bundle branch block the aortic element is delayed, causing either decreased splitting. or even reversed splitting (S_2 tends to close on inspiration) When splitting is present it proves that both semilunar valves are functioning (hence excludes truncus arteriosus, pulmonary atresia or very severe pulmonary stenosis).

Third heart sound (S_3)—a low pitched filling sound due to sudden left ventricular distension, and although normal in children it becomes progressively more unusual with age. It is accentuated when rapid left ventricular filling occurs, e.g. mitral incompetence, ventricular septal defect and patent ductus arteriosus, constrictive pericarditis (here it may be loud enough to be designated a "knock") and left ventricular failure. It is coincident with the peak of the rapid filling wave of the apex cardiogram (see above).

Fourth heart sound (S_4)—heard when atrial systole is more forceful than usual, e.g. right atrial fourth heart sound in pulmonary hypertension, left atrial fourth heart sound in systemic hypertension or aortic stenosis; it is particularly well marked in obstructive cardiomyopathy of the left ventricle (where it often produces a visible and palpable impulse of the apex beat known as presystolic distension).

CARDIAC OUTPUT

This depends on heart rate and stroke volume, which are normally about 70 beats/min. of 70 ml./beat respectively (giving a cardiac output of 4·9 litres/min.). The ventricles do not empty completely with each beat and the total ventricular diastolic volume is about 120 ml. (stroke volume 70 ml., hence residual volume is about 50 ml.).

Stroke volume.—The heart obeys Starling's Law, which states that the energy of contraction is a function of the length of the muscle fibres. Often end-diastolic pressure is used as being equivalent to end-diastolic fibre length although this is only an approximation and probably not always correct. Starling's Law probably applies in man in balancing the outputs of the right and left ventricles and also in the failing heart which has exhausted its noradrenaline reserves. However, under normal conditions the sympathetic nervous system alters the relationships between cardiac work and fibre length such that with an increase in sympathetic discharge more cardiac work is performed for an equivalent myocardial fibre length (Sarnoff has produced a family of Starling curves by varying the amount of sympathetic stimulation of the heart). Hence in health a direct evaluation of Starling's Law for the human heart is difficult to make (can only be done if the sympathetic nervous system is not altered). In man on exercise, there is an increase in cardiac output which is determined by an increase in stroke volume (when the exercise is mild) but with moderate to severe exercise the dominant factor is an increase in heart rate due to an increased sympathetic discharge (there has been confusion in the past regarding the relative increases in heart rate and stroke volume with exercise for, in the supine position, cardiac output increase with exercise is brought about mainly by increasing the heart rate; the previous remarks apply to man exercising in the upright position).

Heart rate.—On reduction of vagus nerve activity together with stimulation of the sympathetic nerves to the heart, the rate of spontaneous depolarisation of the specialised myocardial cells of sino-atrial node is increased and there is a consequent increase in the heart rate. The increase in heart rate is an important determinant of changes in cardiac output under normal circumstances (e.g. the increase in cardiac output in exercise is produced by a tachycardia except at the onset of mild exercise when an increase in stroke volume from approximately 70 ml. to 125 ml. is noted, thereafter an increase in heart rate occurs). In heart failure, with decreased effectiveness of the sympathetic nervous system due to loss of noradrenaline reserves in the heart, there is a greater reliance on increasing myocardial fibre length to increase cardiac output under stress (i.e. dilatation of the heart, whereas in normal individuals the heart becomes smaller with exercise).

METHODS OF DETERMINING CARDIAC OUTPUT

Directly by using a bag enclosing the heart and measuring volume changes with each beat; in man it is possible to determine changes in the size of the heart following thoracotomy if radio-opaque clips are placed on the borders of the heart and serial X-rays taken of the heart.

Fick principle.—The amount of a substance added to or removed from the blood by an organ is equal to the difference between the amount brought into the organ (blood flow through organ × conc. in arterial blood) and the amount carried away (blood flow through organ × conc. in venous blood). In man oxygen is the substance usually measured for determining the cardiac output:

Cardiac output (blood flow through the lungs which is the same as the flow through the left or right ventricle) $= \dfrac{\text{amount of oxygen added to the blood in the lungs}}{\substack{\text{difference between conc. of } O_2 \text{ in blood coming} \\ \text{to and leaving the heart}}}$

Cardiac output $= \dfrac{\text{oxygen consumption (ml./min.)}}{\substack{\text{arteriovenous oxygen content difference across} \\ \text{the lungs (ml./litre blood)}}}$

Dilution techniques, usually using dyes (e.g. indocyanine green); after injection of known amount of dye into the right atrium, arterial blood concentration of the dye is monitored:

Cardiac output $= \dfrac{60 \times \text{amount of dye injected (mg.)}}{\substack{\text{mean conc. of dye (mg./1.)} \times \text{time taken for first} \\ \text{circulation of dye (seconds)}}}$

Cardiac output $= \dfrac{\text{Amount of dye injected}}{\text{Area under dye curve}} \times \text{calibration factor}$

$$= \frac{60.I}{cT}$$

However, radioactive isotopes can be used as indicators, rather than dyes, and measurements made with a precordial scintillation counter (also thermal dilution technique using cold saline as indicator and thermocouples for detection).

Congestive Heart Failure

This is failure of the heart to supply adequately the needs of the tissues for blood leading to the accumulation of blood in the systemic and/or pulmonary circuits. The defect in myocardial contractility may result from:

Incompetence of heart muscle per se—e.g. myocardial infarction with loss of muscle mass; diffuse involvement as in myocarditis or amyloidosis.

Secondary to excessive work load—e.g. valve stenosis or incompetence;

systemic or pulmonary hypertension;

increased blood flow or increased metabolism of body tissues as in Paget's disease of bone, thyrotoxicosis, beri-beri (here causes high output failure where cardiac output may be in excess of that normally seen even though heart failure is present).

Some patients may fall into both groups as in thyrotoxicosis or rheumatic valve lesions where there is often a disorder of cardiac muscle as well as an excessive work load.

The heart consists of two separate muscular pumps, the left and right ventricles, and either pump may fail separately:

left heart failure leads to the accumulation of blood in the pulmonary circuit with rales and dyspnoea (often marked at night and called paroxysmal nocturnal dyspnoea), and often weakness due to low cardiac output; this may progress to congestive heart failure with a clinical picture similar to right heart failure;

right heart failure—systemic engorgement with increased jugular venous pressure, hepatomegaly, ascites and oedema of the ankles.

Starling stated that the energy of cardiac muscle contraction was a function of the length of myocardial muscle fibres; end-diastolic pressure may be taken as an index of fibre length with provisoes (i.e. the higher the end-diastolic pressure the greater the degree of stretching of the muscle fibre). In both high and low output cardiac failure the cardiac output has been found to be consistently lower for any given central venous pressure (which reflects ventricular end-diastolic pressure) than in normal man. Hence one definition of myocardial failure is an abnormal relationship between ventricular work and central venous pressure (illustrated in Figs. 3 and 4 where left atrial pressure reflects left ventricular end-diastolic pressure). It must be reiterated that end-diastolic pressure is used for convenience but does not always represent diastolic fibre length (which is required for a true Starling curve).

The function of the heart is to pump an adequate quantity of blood to the body tissues, and one of the earliest signs of heart failure is inability of the heart to increase cardiac output normally with exercise. Later cardiac output is reduced at rest, the blood pressure being maintained by reflex arteriolar vasoconstriction, which produces reduced blood flow through the skin and splanchnic area; in addition there is a fall in renal blood flow, fall in glomerular filtration rate and retention

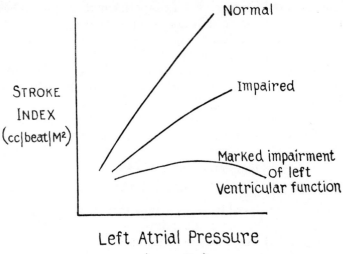

FIG. 3

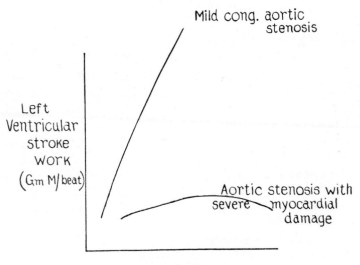

FIG. 4

of sodium (and hence water). In experimental congestive heart failure in dogs with induced pulmonary stenosis, marked sodium retention and ascites occur and there is depressed right ventricular function; unlike some preparations used for studying congestive heart failure, this one responds well to digitalis preparations and appears to satisfy the criteria for congestive heart failure.

The increased renal tubular reabsorption of sodium seen in congestive heart failure (in man and the dog preparation) is due to:

(i) reduced glomerular filtration rate;
(ii) increased blood aldosterone level.

The latter is produced by reduced destruction of aldosterone by the congested liver and by the release of renin from the kidney (see Chapter II) which acts as follows:

```
Reduced afferent arteriolar ──→ Renin release ──→ Angiotensin II ──→ Aldosterone
stretch consequent on           from renal                          release by
diminished myocardial           juxtaglomerular                     adrenal
function          ·             cells                               cortex
```

Support for this hypothesis is provided by reports of increased blood renin and angiotensin levels in congestive heart failure. Increased levels of aldosterone appear rapidly when congestive heart failure is produced in dogs and may occur without measurable fall in glomerular filtration rate, and it is possible that aldosterone release is one of the earliest features of congestive heart failure. There may also be sodium retention primarily due to a fall in glomerular filtration rate alone.

In the treatment of congestive heart failure the following are important:

(i) rest (remember the inability of the heart to increase its output with exercise is an early sign of heart failure);
(ii) digitalis (to increase the efficiency of myocardial contraction);
(iii) reduced salt intake;
(iv) diuretics to increase Na excretion.

PERIPHERAL VASCULAR SYSTEM

The ultimate divisions of the arterial tree are arterioles supplied with smooth muscle under the control of the sympathetic nervous system (and certain humoral materials and metabolites); these vessels regulate the inflow of blood into capillaries which appear without nerve supply and are either fully open or closed, and it is from the capillaries that essential metabolites flow into the interstitial fluid and enter the cells of the tissue.

The resistance to flow in the vascular tree is determined by the calibre of peripheral arterioles on which the sympathetic nervous system exerts a tonic vasoconstrictor influence. Also blood pressure is determined by cardiac output and peripheral vascular resistance:

Blood pressure = Cardiac output × peripheral resistance

$$\text{or C.O.} = \frac{\text{B.P.}}{\text{peripheral resistance}}$$

(modified from Poiseuille's formula). In systemic hypertension the cardiac output is usually normal, hence the increased arterial blood pressure is due to increased peripheral vascular resistance (i.e. hypertension is really a disease of arterioles—see later).

Autonomic vasomotor nerves.—The vasoconstriction normally found in arterioles is due to impulses originating in the vasomotor centre of the medulla. The tonic activity of this centre is modified by impulses arising in baroreceptors in the walls of aorta and carotid sinuses, hence:

an increase in — stimulates baroreceptors — feedback to — reduced
arterial   vasomotor   vasocon-
pressure   centre   strictor
                                                                tone
                                                                  |
reduces blood pressure — lowers peripheral — relaxes arteriolar wall
                         resistance

These nerves provide rapid adjustment of the circulation to changing flows and pressures. Only certain parts of the circulation take part in these adjustments of peripheral resistance, particularly the splanchnic circulation and the skin. The vasomotor centre is acted on by impulses from higher centres, e.g. cerebral cortex, hypothalamus temperature-regulating centre.

NERVOUS CONTROL OF BLOOD VESSELS

Sympathetic vasoconstrictors.—Centre (vasomotor centre) in the medulla; they cause constriction of arterioles and are all adrenergic (i.e. liberate noradrenaline at their terminations on smooth muscle cells of arterioles).

Vasodilator fibres.—Sympathetic—active vasodilatation can be produced by sympathetic cholinergic fibres (i.e. liberate acetylcholine at their endings), e.g. to muscle blood vessels and to skin (in the latter case bradykinin, a nonapeptide, is produced which causes vasodilatation in skin and also salivary glands).

Vasodilator fibres.—Parasympathetic—cholinergic and of limited distribution, especially to pelvic viscera (e.g. erection).

Vasodilatation brought about for the purpose of blood pressure regulation is the result of variations in constrictor activity (the cholinergic vasodilator fibres play no part in this). Local increase in blood flow for specific organ function may be brought about by other mechanisms (e.g. cholinergic fibres, either sympathetic or parasympathetic, bradykinin, local metabolites, etc.).

HUMORAL CONTROL OF BLOOD VESSELS

The products of *local metabolism*, e.g. carbon dioxide, adenosine monophosphate (AMP) can cause vasodilatation and may be of importance in reactive hyperaemia or, in the case of AMP, may control the coronary circulation in response to an increased work load by the heart.

Circulating in the blood stream are *humoral materials*, e.g. angiotensin, a powerful vasoconstrictor (present in the blood in malignant hypertension), adrenaline, noradrenaline (causes hypertension due to its constricting effect on the peripheral arterioles; secreted in excess in phaeochromocytoma—see Chapter II), and other vasoactive materials.

It is germane in this section to study the α and β receptors. This concept arose when attempts were made to explain the action of adrenaline which causes contraction of some smooth muscle (e.g. in arterioles in most parts of the body) and relaxation of smooth muscle in other areas (e.g. smooth muscle in blood vessels in skeletal muscle). α receptors are in vascular smooth muscle involved in constriction under the influence of adrenaline while β receptors respond by vasodilation. β receptors are also responsible for increasing the rate and strength of cardiac contraction and relaxation of bronchial smooth muscle, and may be specifically blocked by propranolol, while α receptors are responsible for vasoconstriction, intestinal relaxation, glycogenolysis, etc. and can be blocked by Dibenzyline.

Hypertension.—Pulmonary hypertension is considered below: systemic (diastolic) hypertension is essentially a persistent elevation of peripheral vascular resistance (which is an important determinant of diastolic blood pressure). Hypertension may be arbitrarily be taken as a persistent elevation of diastolic blood pressure, the pathological limit being determined by age and there is no sharp dividing line between normal and abnormal blood pressure. (So-called systolic hypertension, i.e. elevation of systolic arterial blood pressure only, with essentially normal diastolic values, is due either to increased stroke output, e.g. thyrotoxicosis, or reduced distensibility of the blood vessels, e.g. arteriosclerosis; it is not usually treated).

The causes of systemic diastolic hypertension are often divided into known (secondary hypertension) and unknown (primary or essential hypertension):

Primary essential hypertension.

Secondary to:

(i) renal disease, e.g. acute and chronic nephritis, renal artery stenosis (hypertension possibly initiated by renin release);

(ii) adrenal cortical dysfunction, e.g. mainly excess mineralocorticoids (Conn's syndrome), or glucocorticoids and mineralocorticoids (Cushing's syndrome) (see Chapter II);

(iii) adrenal medullary dysfunction, e.g. phaeochromocytoma (producing excess catecholamine release—see Chapter II);

(iv) obstruction to flow, e.g. coarctation of the aorta;

(v) toxaemia of pregnancy;

(vi) neurogenic hypertension—removal of feed-back mechanisms from baroreceptors in the carotid sinus and aortic body can produce peripheral vasoconstriction and hence hypertension in experimental animals; the importance in man is not clear.

The malignant phase of hypertension is a rapidly progressive (accelerated) form of hypertension with increased renin release and arteriolar necrosis from the stress of the high arterial pressure.

The response of the peripheral vascular bed to various stimuli (the vascular reactivity) is altered in certain diseases (e.g. increased blood pressure rise in certain people with a stressful stimulus who later develop hypertension, the so-called pre-hypertensive patient). There is no doubt that the state of the peripheral vascular tree is influenced by its water and electrolyte content which is of importance when considering the treatment of hypertension.

PHYSIOLOGICAL BACKGROUND TO TREATMENT OF HYPERTENSION

The aim of therapy is to reduce the total peripheral resistance to blood flow by:

(a) altering smooth muscle activity directly;
(b) reducing nervous or neurogenic vasoconstriction.

The drugs employed are:

Diuretics—reduce amount of sodium (and hence water) in the body, but besides causing a fall in blood volume, they reduce the peripheral resistance.

Rauwolfia alkaloids—reduce noradrenaline content of sympathetic nerve endings to blood vessels, i.e. impair adrenergic transmission, reduce peripheral resistance and hence lower blood pressure.

Guanethidine—selectively inhibits adrenergic neurone transmission by preventing release of noradrenaline at the termination of nerve fibres on vascular smooth muscle cells.

Methyldopa—produces noradrenaline depletion at sympathetic nerve endings on vascular smooth muscle cells possibly by producing an α-methyl noradrenaline to replace noradrenaline; this makes transmission much less effective, hence reducing peripheral resistance and lowering arterial blood pressure.

Elevation of blood pressure increases the work of the myocardium, which may fail if the hypertension is of long standing, and often this occurs in the presence of inadequate perfusion of the coronary arteries due to vascular disease (atherosclerosis) partly produced by the prolonged increased blood pressure.

Shock

A syndrome whose central feature is an overall insufficiency of blood flow. Conventionally divisible into:

Primary or neurogenic shock—e.g. vasovagal attack (a faint) in which vagal bradycardia occurs together with dilatation of muscle blood vessels.

In this the genesis is as follows:

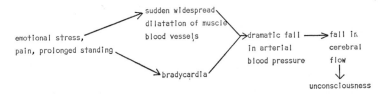

Secondary shock.—This may be due to blood or plasma loss, loss of fluids and electrolytes, overwhelming infection, coronary thrombosis; although the various causes of the above lead to a similar clinical picture the mechanisms responsible are *not* the same.

Haemorrhagic shock.—This is the easiest example of shock to understand:

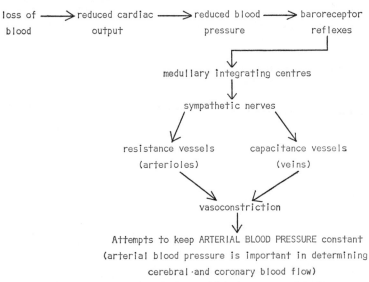

It is this intense vasoconstriction which is responsible for many of the clinical features of shock; it also leads to tissue damage because of tissue hypoxia. In spite of these various compensatory mechanisms, blood pressure may fall and probably the final stage of irreversible shock is due to tissue damage and failure of the myocardium to pump adequately.

The clinical picture is dependent on the intense vasoconstriction produced:

   (i) reduced blood flow to skin—pale skin;
  (ii) increased sympathetic activity—clammy skin and increased heart rate;
 (iii) reduced blood flow to salivary glands—dry mouth and thirst;
 (iv) reduced blood flow to intestines—impaired digestion and reduced water absorption;
  (v) reduced blood flow to kidneys—fall in urine output.

Compensation for blood loss depends on:

 (a) Starling's Law of capillaries—as hydrostatic pressure falls the osmotic pressure exerted by the plasma proteins withdraws fluid from interstitial space and puts it into the circulating fluid compartment (see Chapter IV);
 (b) Loss of plasma proteins is restored by synthesis in liver;
 (c) Red cell loss is replaced by the action of released erythropoietin on bone marrow.

Hence in the treatment of shock adequate fluid replacement is mandatory (e.g. blood, dextran, etc.), but tissue perfusion, of which blood pressure is an inadequate measure, is probably the essential key to shock and its reversibility (which accounts for the efficacy of some vasodilators in shock).

Mechanisms in other types of shock probably are as follows:

Traumatic shock—loss of circulating fluid + toxins from damaged tissues + infection.

Septic shock—variable pathogenesis, e.g. toxins in anthrax septicaemia in the guinea-pig lead to oedema and hypovolaemic shock.

Burn shock—loss of circulating fluid (plasma) and heat destruction of red cells.

Cardiogenic shock—inadequacy of the myocardial pump.

BLOOD FLOW IN SPECIAL CIRCUITS

Pulmonary Circulation

This receives the total cardiac output but the pressure is only about 1/5th of the systemic pressure, hence it is a low resistance circuit (with a large capacity). There is little, if any, influence on it from the nervous system, no tonic vasoconstrictor tone of note, and hypoxia is the only potent vasoconstrictor. Pulmonary arterial pressure depends upon the output of right ventricle and the resistance to blood flow through the pulmonary vessels, and normally is about 30/15 mm.Hg. Elevated pulmonary artery pressure (pulmonary hypertension) may be due to an increase in pulmonary vascular resistance (e.g. severe emphysema, recurrent pulmonary thrombo-embolism, collagen diseases, sarcoidosis, bilharzia and finally idiopathic causes). The rise in pulmonary artery pressure in mitral stenosis is sometimes due to vasoconstriction but is often merely a reflection of elevated left atrial pressure.

Cerebral Circulation

Cerebral blood flow is determined by:

Cerebral autoregulation—there is a tendency for cerebral blood flow to remain relatively constant in the face of changing pressures due to constriction of arterioles when systemic pressure increases, and vice versa (known as *autoregulation*); this fails when the arterial pressure is too low and cerebral blood flow then falls;

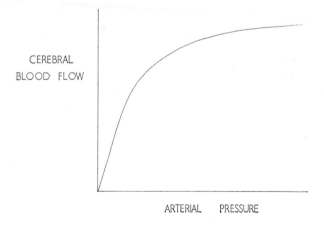

CEREBRAL
BLOOD FLOW

ARTERIAL   PRESSURE

Effective perfusion pressure—arterial blood pressure is the sole determinant of the driving force of blood flow across the brain;

Cerebral vascular resistance—the nervous system has little effect on cerebral vascular resistance, and carbon dioxide is the most powerful cerebral vasodilator known.

Hence, like the pulmonary vascular tree, there is a lack of effective vasomotor regulation by the autonomic nervous system, the main determinants of flow being the cerebral autoregulating mechanism, arterial blood pressure and chemical control of vascular resistance (essentially carbon dioxide only).

Coronary Circulation

A large fraction of the oxygen supplied in the blood from the coronary arteries is extracted by the heart (therefore for the myocardium to obtain more oxygen under stress coronary blood flow must increase). The main factor determining flow is again the arterial blood pressure (the driving force across the coronary bed) and changes in vessel calibre are probably produced by metabolites rather than any direct nervous influence on the coronary bed. Increase in myocardial work causes increased coronary flow due to local tissue hypoxia probably, so that myocardial oxygen utilisation is the main determinant of coronary flow (besides arterial blood pressure), a possible controlling mechanism being:

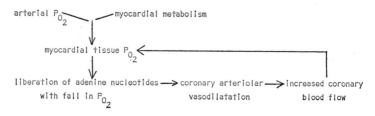

Chapter IV

pH, FLUID AND ELECTROLYTE BALANCE

THE gram-equivalent of an atom, molecule or ion is that weight which combines with or displaces 1 g. of hydrogen ion in a reaction. For a monovalent ion this is the same as the ionic weight, for a divalent ion it is half its ionic weight. In biological solutions a thousandth part or milli-equivalent (mEq.) is the conventional unit.

The concentration of hydrogen ions $[H^+]$ and the concentration of hydroxyl ions $[OH^-]$ in a solution in water is constant (for any given temperature). At 23°C

$$[H^+] = 10^{-7} \text{ gram equivalents/litre}$$
$$= 0 \cdot 0000001 \text{ mole H/litre.}$$

On the pH notation,

$$pH = -\log_{10} [H^+]$$

(p means that the negative logarithm, to base 10, is used instead of the quantity itself).

In pure water at 23°C $[H^+] = 0 \cdot 0000001 = 10^{-7}$.

As $pH = -\log_{10} [H^+]$, the pH of pure water at 23°C is 7·0 (in pure water at 38°C pH = 6·8).

The reaction of a solution is called acid when the concentration of hydrogen ions in it is greater than the concentration of hydroxyl ions (vice versa for alkaline solutions). In pure water $[H^+] = [OH^-]$ and the reaction is neutral, and from the above pH = 7.

The reaction of the plasma of arterial blood in healthy people is pH 7·36 to 7·44, corresponding to a $[H^+]$ of 0·00004 ± 0·000004 mEq/litre. The pH of pure water (neutral) at 38°C is 6·8, hence the reaction of arterial blood is on the alkaline side of neutrality. Reasonable stability of pH is a necessary requirement for survival of man and this is accomplished by buffers in the blood. The most important **buffers** are:

haemoglobin in erythrocytes

$\left.\begin{array}{l} \textit{bicarbonate} \\ \textit{protein} \\ \textit{phosphate} \end{array}\right\}$ *in the plasma*

A buffer solution is one which can accommodate the addition to it of moderate amounts of acid (which is a molecule or ion with a tendency to lose a proton) or base (tendency to take up protons) without marked change in its hydrogen ion concentration [H+], e.g. salt of weak acid and strong base (HB) which in solution dissociates:

$$HB \rightleftharpoons H^+ + B^-.$$

If the pH falls, the increasing concentration of H+ ion displaces the equilibrium towards the left, i.e. favours the reaction which removes H+ from the solution (and vice versa).

The most important buffer anion (or H+ acceptor) in blood is the haemoglobin ion (due to the dissociation of imidazole groups of histidine in the haemoglobin molecule); the plasma proteins act as hydrogen acceptors (the buffering power is much less than that of haemoglobin, being approximately 1/6th that of the total haemoglobin). The reactions for the buffering of H+ by these buffer anions are:

$$H^+ + HCO_3^- \rightarrow H_2CO_3 \ (\rightarrow CO_2 + H_2O)$$
$$H^+ + HPO_4^= \rightarrow H_2PO_4^-$$
$$H^+ + Protein^- \rightarrow H \ Protein$$

in general terms:

$$H^+ + Buffer^- \rightleftharpoons HBuf.$$

In the buffer solution of bicarbonate and carbonic acid the general equation of Henderson-Hasselbalch applies:

$$pH = pK + Log\frac{[HCO_3^-]}{[H_2CO_3]} \text{ and } pK = 6 \cdot 1$$

The solubility of carbon dioxide in water at $37°C = 0 \cdot 033$ × partial pressure of CO_2 (P_{CO_2} in mm.Hg). If partial pressure of carbon dioxide (P_{CO_2}) = 40 mm.Hg, then $[CO_2]$ at equilibrium = $40 \times 0 \cdot 033$ = approx. $1 \cdot 35$ mMole/litre while $[HCO_3^-]$ is 27 mEq/litre water.

Now H_2CO_3 is in equilibrium with dissolved carbon dioxide

$$H_2CO_3 \rightleftharpoons H_2O + CO_2.$$

Hence the Henderson-Hasselbalch equation can be rewritten as:

$$pH = 6 \cdot 1 + \log \frac{27}{1 \cdot 35} = 6 \cdot 1 + \log 20 = 6 \cdot 1 + 1 \cdot 3 = 7 \cdot 4$$

or else

$$pH = 6 \cdot 1 + \log \frac{[HCO_3^-]}{P_{CO_2} \times 0 \cdot 033}.$$

In practice pH, $[HCO_3^-]$ and P_{CO_2} can be measured, hence the knowledge of any two enables the third to be calculated.

THE REGULATION OF pH

Buffer systems within the body—cellular, e.g. haemoglobin extracellular, e.g. bicarbonate, protein, phosphate buffers.
Respiratory regulation of carbon dioxide excretion.
Renal regulation of hydrogen ion excretion.

Respiratory Regulation of Carbon Dioxide Concentration

Carbon dioxide is the end-product of many metabolic processes:

$$CO_2 + H_2O \rightleftharpoons H_2CO_3 \rightleftharpoons H^+ + HCO_3^-$$

Carbon dioxide is removed by the lungs and the above reaction moves from right to left and hydrogen ions, originally formed in the tissues, disappear (the excretion of carbon dioxide depends on the P_{CO_2} of alveolar air which determines the P_{CO_2} in arterial blood to the respiratory centre in the medulla). Hydrogen ions are not excreted by the lungs, but any change in the elimination of carbon dioxide will alter the pH of the body fluids by altering the P_{CO_2}. Note the size of the pulmonary excretion of carbon dioxide compared with the renal excretion of hydrogen ion: normal subject excretes 15,000 mEq (300 litres) carbon dioxide daily through the lungs; 50 mEq hydrogen daily through kidneys (max. 600 mEq daily).

Renal Regulation of Hydrogen Ion Excretion

Strong acids ingested or formed by metabolic reactions account for the production of about 50 mEq. H^+ daily (especially derived from sulphuric and phosphoric acids formed by protein metabolism), which must be excreted by the kidneys. Originally these acids combine with buffer bases in the extra-cellular fluid, reducing the amount of buffer available while not changing the pH of the extracellular fluid. The kidney has to restore the buffering capacity of the body by excreting H^+ which it does by generating and excreting new H^+ in the urine (excreted in exchange for Na^+ reabsorbed from the urine) (see Chapter IX).

The kidney regulates pH by:

excreting excess HCO_3^- from the body in the urine (e.g. during a metabolic alkalosis);

excreting H^+ ion (produced inside the tubular cells by the enzyme, carbonic anhydrase) in exchange for Na^+ (which is reabsorbed from the urine) or K^+.

   (i) H^+ ion excreted in combination with ammonia produced in renal tubular cells;
   (ii) H^+ ion excreted in combination with phosphate present in tubular fluid.

The method by which the renal tubules make the urine acid by directly secreting H^+ into it will be dealt with in the chapter on The Kidney.

CLINICAL DISORDERS OF pH REGULATION

Respiratory acidosis.—Usually due to hypoventilation causing a primary increase in blood P_{CO_2}; the kidney compensates by excreting more H^+ and retaining HCO_3^-, but can only com-pensate in chronic, not acute, respiratory acidosis because of its limited capacity to excrete H^+.

Respiratory alkalosis.—Primary change is a reduction of alveolar P_{CO_2} due to hyperventilation; kidney compensates by excreting more HCO_3^-.

Metabolic acidosis.—Increased ingestion or production of acids, other than carbonic acid, in the extracellular fluid, e.g. excess production of acids in diabetic ketosis, reduced excretion of organic acids in chronic renal failure, or failure to excrete H^+ due to a congenital defect of the renal tubular cells. The primary change is a fall in plasma $[HCO_3^-]$ and pH, and the lungs compensate by blowing off carbon dioxide.

Metabolic alkalosis.—Decreased concentration of acids, other than carbonic, in the extracellular fluid, e.g. loss of acid in the persistent vomiting of pyloric stenosis or increased ingestion of alkali (such as sodium bicarbonate taken orally as therapy for peptic ulcer). Primary change is an increase in the plasma [HCO_3^-] and the kidney compensates by excreting HCO_3^-.

For purposes of simplicity the Henderson-Hasselbalch equation may be presented as follows (Robinson's *Fundamentals of Acid-Base Regulation*, 1965, p. 23, by kind permission).

$$pH = pK + \log \frac{\text{kidneys}}{\text{lungs and respiratory centre}}$$

BODY FLUIDS

Volume.—In an average 70 kg. person, there is about 45 litres of water (about 65 per cent by weight in the normal adult male, but less in obese individuals). Total body water can be determined by using antipyrine, deuterium oxide ("heavy water") or tritium oxide using the dilution principle. The body water is divided into two main compartments:

intracellular fluid (approx. 70 per cent total body water or 45 – 50 per cent body weight);

extracellular fluid (approx. 30 per cent total body water or 12 – 15 per cent body weight; about 12 litres).

(*a*) Extravascular or interstitial fluid (lies outside blood vessels and between tissue cells; approx. 9 litres);

(*b*) intravascular or plasma water (approx. 3 litres in the vascular space).

The plasma volume (approx. 3 litres) is smaller than the blood volume which includes the red cells (volume approx. 5 litres); the blood volume is about 70 ml./kg. while plasma volume is about 45 ml./kg. body weight. The plasma volume is determined by dilution techniques using either dyes (e.g. Evans blue) or radio-isotopes (radioactive iodinated human serum albumin, RIHSA).

Composition.—The body fluids differ greatly in their composition:

intracellular fluid—contains protein; main cation K^+, main anions HPO_4^-, $SO_4^=$ and protein$^-$.

extracellular fluid—very little K^+ and main cation Na^+; main anions Cl^- and HCO_3^-.

The interstitial and intravascular fluids are of almost identical composition except for a much larger protein content in the latter (6 – 8 G./100 ml., see Chapter V).

K^+—about 3400 mEq. in the body, 95 per cent intracellular and remainder in the extracellular fluid (ECF) at a concentration of 4·5 mEq/1.

Na^+—about 4000 mEq. in the body, large amount is present in the bones; about 400 mEq. intracellular (concentration 15 mEq/1.) while 1600 mEq. in ECF (concentration about 140 mEq/1.). The maintenance of the extracellular position of Na^+ depends on the active extrusion of the ion from inside cells by a "sodium pump" (see Chapter X).

Water Balance

Water is lost from body by:

the lungs—approx. 400 cc./24 hours normally;

faeces—normally 200 ml. daily, but greatly increased in severe diarrhoea, e.g. cholera where the course of the disease is largely determined by water and electrolyte loss in the faeces;

skin (i) insensible perspiration;
　　　(ii) sweating.

Water loss through the skin is very variable depending on bodily activity, amount of clothing, temperature, humidity and circulation of the surrounding air. In a temperate climate the loss is about 500 – 1000 ml./24 hours (but an individual can lose up to 900 ml./hr. when working in a hot humid environment). As there is only a small salt content in sweat, the loss is largely water, and the loss of sweat cannot be controlled by the water-regulating mechanism of the body.

Urine—by altering water loss through the kidneys the water content of the body is controlled (see Chapter IX). Urine is necessary for the removal of various end-products of metabolism (especially urea), and as the maximum urinary concentrating power of the kidney can produce a urine with an osmolarity of 1300 milliosmols/litre (equivalent to a specific gravity of about 1·035), the daily solute load can be excreted in no less than about 500 ml. of urine. If the effective water intake is very low, the water available to the kidneys for excretion of solute is reduced—there is a fall in urine flow and an increase in the blood urea concentration (e.g. cholera). If the concentrating power of the kidneys falls, the minimum obligatory urine volume has to increase if the same amount of solute is to be excreted (e.g. chronic nephritis). The total minimum daily water loss from the body is about 1500 ml., and the intake must equal this (ingested food and liquids + water derived from the oxidation of the food) for equilibrium to be maintained.

CONTROL OF WATER BALANCE

Factors controlling intake—thirst.

Factors controlling excretion—posterior pituitary antidiuretic hormone (see Chapter IX).

Antidiuretic hormone is secreted in response to an increase in osmolarity of the blood, which is detected by hypothalamic osmoreceptors which lead to release of ADH which acts on the distal and collecting tubules of the nephron to increase their permeability to water (and hence increase reabsorption of water and concentrate the urine) (see Chapter IX).

CONTROL OF Na^+ BALANCE

Control of Na^+ excretion is less well understood and it is Na^+ which is primarily responsible for the volume of the extracellular fluid (while water excretion determines its osmolarity). Acute changes in glomerular filtration rate alter Na^+ excretion (a reduction in glomerular filtration rate increases tubular sodium reabsorption), e.g. reduced glomerular filtration rate in hypovolaemic shock due to loss causes increased Na^+ reabsorption, and hence water retention, in an attempt to restore the *status quo* with respect to ECF volume. Increased tubular Na^+ retention is produced by aldosterone from the adrenal cortex, the stimulus being reduced renal blood flow and/or reduced pulse pressure (causing renin release and consequent aldosterone production; see Chapter II). There are other mechanisms involved in long continued Na^+ retention for this cannot be produced by the long-term administration of aldosterone as there is an "escape" from the sodium-retaining effects of this hormone (possibly due to a humoral factor from outside the adrenal gland which sensitises the renal tubular cells to the sodium-retaining action of aldosterone).

CLINICAL DISORDERS OF Na^+ AND WATER METABOLISM

Water depletion—e.g. stranded in the desert, adrift at sea. There is a diminution in ECF volume and a rise in its osmolarity, and water passes from the intracellular to the extracellular phase. At first thirst, dry mouth and tongue occur, followed later by delirium, coma and death. The urine is concentrated and it contains a high concentration of electrolytes and urea; later there is a rise in the blood urea level.

Na^+ depletion—e.g. excessive sweating with replacement of water only. There is a fall in osmolarity of the ECF, some water is excreted by the kidney while some moves intracellularly, and the final result is a fall in ECF volume. In the early stages the patient is lethargic and has diminished skin elasticity, while later there is more marked weakness with postural faintness, then a rising pulse rate and falling blood pressure and low cardiac output (a clinical picture of "shock"), muscle cramps often occur, as does nausea and vomiting. The urine contains negligible amounts of Na^+ and is moderately concentrated; the ECF volume falls and there is a rise in haematocrit (not seen in the *early* stages of water depletion where ECF volume remains normal on account of the compensatory shift of intracellular water); later there is a fall in renal blood flow which causes a rise in blood urea concentration.

Mixed type of sodium and water depletion seen in clinical practice is most commonly due to abnormal losses of intestinal secretions (vomiting, diarrhoea or external fistula) which causes water (intracellular) and sodium (extracellular) depletion. The clinical picture may show thirst, sparse urine (little or no sodium in it), increased haematocrit and blood urea. Infants are particularly sensitive to fluid depletion (the daily turnover of fluid may be as high as one half of their ECF whereas in adults the comparable loss would only amount to about one seventh of the ECF).

K^+ Balance

Intake—by mouth.

Output—in urine and from the gastro-intestinal tract; potassium balance is maintained by aldosterone (which promotes its excretion in the urine).

CLINICAL DISORDERS OF K⁺ BALANCE

Hypokalaemia—weakness and paralysis of skeletal muscle, intestinal ileus, apathy. Due to shift of K^+ into cells in the treatment of uncontrolled diabetes with acidosis, excessive loss in diarrhoea, primary aldosteronism and Cushing's syndrome, and also due to prolonged diuretic therapy.

Hyperkalaemia—muscle paralysis and serious ECG changes (also seen in hypokalaemia). Due to renal failure, severe injuries to tissues which release the intracellular K^+.

[See Chapter II for details of **Calcium metabolism**]

Oedema.—Fluid exchange between plasma and interstitial fluid occurs due to:

(a) difference between capillary blood pressure and interstitial fluid pressure;

(b) difference between plasma protein and interstitial fluid protein osmotic pressure.

The essential mechanisms involved in Starling's Law of Capillaries are summarised in Fig. 5. The lymphatics are vessels which ramify in the tissues and drain off excess interstitial fluid.

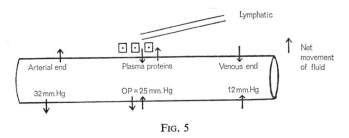

FIG. 5

Oedema is the excessive accumulation of fluid in the interstitial space which may be due to local or general disturbance of the circulation of interstitial fluid. The following mechanisms may apply:

1. Increased venous pressure, e.g. prolonged standing (influence of gravity on local venous pressure in the legs).

2. Decrease in tissue tension opposing hydrostatic pressure, e.g. famine oedema.

3. Obstruction to lymphatic drainage, e.g. in arm after radical mastectomy, fibrosis of the lymphatic channels due to certain parasites as in filariasis.
4. Excess reabsorption of sodium, e.g. in the oedema of congestive heart failure.
5. Decreased plasma osmotic pressure due to reduction in plasma protein concentration, e.g. renal loss of albumin in nephrotic syndrome, famine oedema.
6. Increased capillary permeability to plasma proteins, e.g. inflammation, urticaria.

The formation of oedema in any patient may depend on more than one of the above mechanisms.

Chapter V

BLOOD

THERE are three formed elements, the red cells, white cells (leucocytes) and platelets suspended in a fluid, plasma. These cells are being continually manufactured and destroyed; the sites of formation are:

red cells—bone marrow;
white cells—lymphocytes, monocytes—lymph nodes and
                    other collections of lymphoid tissue;
            —granular leucocytes—bone marrow;
platelets—bone marrow.

RED CELLS

Manufacture of red cells.—A major factor controlling the rate of production is the arterial oxygen content (really the tissue oxygen pressure or P_{O_2}). This action may not be a direct one on the bone marrow but rather via the hormone erythropoietin (see Chapter II). The endocrine organs also play some part in the regulation of erythropoiesis e.g. reduction of red cell count in eunuchoid males is reversed by androgens, the anaemia of myxoedema, etc.

The red cell is composed of an outer envelope of lipoprotein complexed with the protein of the stroma, the latter containing a concentrated solution of haemoglobin. Haemoglobin is composed of a molecule of the protein globin to which is attached 4 molecules of haem (haem = protoporphyrin + ferrous iron), and has a molecular weight of 68,000. The red cell maintains its functional integrity by two main metabolic activities:

(i) anaerobic glycolysis via the Embden-Meyerhof pathway (see Chapter I), and the energy from this is used to maintain the integrity of the cell membrane and the selective exchange of ions across it;

(ii) the hexose monophosphate shunt (which supplies reduced nicotinamide adenine dinucleotide phosphate, $NADPH_2$ formerly TPNH, for the reduction of glutathione and hence prevents the oxidative degradation of haemoglobin to methaemoglobin).

There are a large number of substances necessary for erythropoiesis, some come from the metabolic pool of the body and others are specific factors for red cell production e.g. aminoacids, Fe, vitamin B_{12}, folic acid, trace metals, etc.

Normally there are $4\cdot5 - 6\cdot5$ million red cells/cubic mm. blood in adult man and the haemoglobin concentration is $13\cdot5 - 18\cdot0$ G./100 ml. blood with a packed cell volume (haematocrit) of $40 - 54$ per cent, and a mean corpuscular haemoglobin concentration (MCHC = Hb in G./100 ml. ÷ packed cell volume and expressed as a percentage) of $32 - 36$ per cent.

Destruction of red cells.—Average life span $100 - 120$ days, and as red cells grow older their enzyme systems probably fail making them more susceptible to phagocytosis by reticuloendothelial cells. Inside the phagocytic cells haemoglobin is released and the protein globin is split off from the haem which is then broken down to iron and porphyrin. The porphyrin is broken down in the phagocyte to bilirubin which passes into the plasma (forming a loose complex with albumin) and is removed from the circulation by the parenchymal cells of the liver and excreted in the bile (see Chapter VIII).

BLOOD GROUPS

Human red cells contain on their surface a series of blood group antigens which are genetically controlled, the main ones being of the ABO system, e.g.

group AB cells possess both A and B antigen;
group A cells possess only A antigen;
group O cells have neither antigen on their surfaces.

The plasma of an individual contains antibodies against the antigens lacking in his red cells, e.g.

group A person has anti-B agglutinins in his plasma, so that his plasma will cause group B red cells to clump together.

Rhesus blood groups.—First demonstrated on human red cells using an antiserum prepared by immunizing rabbits with injections of blood from the Rhesus monkey. Some human red cells were agglutinated by this serum—i.e. Rh positive cells.

These blood groups are important in medicine in:

 (i) haemolytic transfusion reactions;
 (ii) haemolytic disease of the newborn (usually due to Rh incompatibility between foetus and mother).

ANAEMIA

This is a reduction in the concentration of haemoglobin in the peripheral blood below the normal for the age and sex of the patient. There are a variety of compensatory physiological adjustments to counteract the reduction in oxygen carrying capacity of the blood (e.g. increased cardiac output, increased plasma volume, increased oxygen utilisation by the tissues). The clinical picture of the anaemic patient will depend on the degree of anaemia and rate of production and age of the patient, and the disorder primarily responsible for the anaemia.

Anaemia results from three fundamental disturbances:

 (*a*) blood loss;
 (*b*) impaired red cell formation;
 (*c*) excess red cell destruction.

Blood Loss

This may be either acute or chronic, the latter usually causing a normocytic normochromic anaemia until the body's iron stores are exhausted when the red cells become smaller with less haemoglobin content (microcytic hypochromic anaemia). The major causes of iron deficiency anaemia in men and post-menopausal females is pathological blood loss, while in females in the reproductive period it is menstruation and pregnancy. Although the great majority of hypochromic anaemias are due to iron deficiency there are a number of disorders in which hypochromic anaemia is not due to iron deficiency (non-sideropoenic hypochromic anaemias) e.g. anaemia of infection, of rheumatoid arthritis, renal insufficiency, disseminated malignancy, etc.

Impaired Red Cell Formation

 (i) *Disturbance of bone marrow function either "metabolic" or due to infiltration with abnormal cells.*—E.g. infection, renal disease, disseminated malignancy, aplastic anaemia, malignant lymphomas, myelosclerosis, etc.

Note that from the above it will be seen that more than one factor may be responsible for the anaemia in certain clinical states.

In aplastic anaemia there is a reduction in the amount of haemopoietic bone marrow and insufficient number of mature cells are discharged into the circulation. May be:

Primary—no known cause.

Secondary—due to the toxic action of *chemicals and drugs*, drugs used in the treatment of malignant lymphomas and leukaemias e.g. nitrogen mustard; an abnormal reaction to a drug e.g. anti-epileptic drugs, phenylbutazone, gold salts, chloramphenicol; industrial chemicals e.g. benzene and its derivatives, paraphenylenediamine; due to *physical agents* e.g. X-rays, radioactive materials.

(ii) *Disturbance of bone marrow function due to deficiency of substances essential for erythropoiesis.*

> I   Fe
> II Vitamin B_{12}
> III Folic acid

Iron is present in haemoglobin, in the plasma (bound to a beta globulin, siderophilin) and in the tissues (essential, non-available iron as in myoglobin and cytochromes, and in available, storage form as the soluble ferritin and the insoluble form, haemosiderin). The serum iron value is about 120 micro-grams/100 ml. Iron is present in the food mainly in the ferric state and as various complexes, but it is mainly, but not exclusively, absorbed in the ionic (ferrous) form, mainly in the duodenum. The control of absorption is related to the size of the iron stores and the rate of erythropoiesis (the exact mechanism is unknown although recent work again confirms that the mucosal cells control it to some extent). In haemochromatosis there is massive iron accumulation in the liver and there is some genetic evidence for this being due to increased iron absorption possibly with additional liver damage from alcohol or virus infection (i.e. excess iron absorption may not be the sole determinant).

Deficiency of vitamin B_{12} or folic acid can cause a mega-loblastic anaemia (the anaemia is macrocytic i.e. mean corpus-cular volume over the maximum normal volume of 96 c.μ., and it is associated with abnormal red cell precursors in the bone marrow called megaloblasts). 90 per cent of megaloblastic anaemias (in temperate climates) are of the Addisonian type while the remainder are usually associated with gastro-intestinal disorders (ranging from sprue, anatomical lesions of the intestine, to infestation with fish tapeworm), defective nutrition, pregnancy and anticonvulsant therapy.

Vitamin B$_{12}$ acts as a co-enzyme in reactions leading to nucleic acid synthesis and is essential for normal erythropoiesis and maintenance of the integrity of the nervous system. Its absorption from foodstuffs in the terminal ileum is facilitated by intrinsic factor (a mucoprotein secreted in man by mucosal cells of the fundus and cardia of the stomach), and it is stored in the liver. Deficiency is nearly always due to some disorder of the alimentary tract:

(a) lack of intrinsic factor (Addisonian pernicious anaemia; gastric atrophy, total gastrectomy, 6 per cent of partial gastrectomy patients);

(b) interference by bacteria or parasites with normal absorption of B$_{12}$ e.g. stagnation in a blind loop of gut, fish tapeworm, fistula by-passing terminal ileum;

(c) interference with the absorptive capacity of the intestinal mucosa e.g. idiopathic steatorrhoea, tropical sprue.

There are three clinical manifestations of vitamin B$_{12}$ deficiency of whatever aetiology:

(i) megaloblastic macrocytic anaemia;

(ii) glossitis;

(iii) peripheral neuritis and subacute combined degeneration of the spinal cord.

Folic acid is absorbed in the jejunum and is also essential for normal erythropoiesis and for normal nucleic acid synthesis, particularly the desoxyribose nucleic acid (DNA) of the cell nucleus; it is necessary for the mucosal cells of the alimentary tract (hence deficiency in man leads to glossitis, anorexia, diarrhoea).

Deficiency results from:

inadequate intake (often together with pregnancy);
intestinal malabsorption (e.g. coeliac disease);

increased demand (e.g. pregnancy);
inability to utilise it because of folic acid antagonists (e.g. anticonvulsant therapy).

There are two important clinical manifestations:

macrocytic megaloblastic anaemia;
glossitis.
No nervous system manifestations.

There is also a heterogeneous group of macrocytic anaemias with a *normoblastic* bone marrow (e.g. haemolytic anaemias, acute leukaemias, anaemias due to bone marrow replacement or infiltration).

Excess red cell destruction.—A haemolytic anaemia is due to an increased rate of red cell destruction (normal red cell life span of 120 days is reduced). There are two fundamental causes:

1. *Intrinsic* (*intracorpuscular*) *abnormality* of the red cells which renders them more susceptible to the normal mechanisms of cell destruction:

    (i) due to an inherent metabolic defect e.g. hereditary spherocytosis (familial acholuric jaundice) where the cells have an abnormal shape;
    (ii) due to the presence of an abnormal form of haemoglobin, either due to the inhibition of normal adult Hb formation (thalassaemia or Cooley's anaemia) or the production of an abnormal variant of Hb e.g. sickle cell anaemia (the Hb assumes an elongated shape at reduced blood oxygen tensions and this disrupts the cell membrane causing haemolysis and the abnormal erythrocytes block capillaries causing small areas of infarction in many tissues). Although the mechanism of the intrinsic abnormality is unclear in most instances, in hereditary spherocytosis the primary abnormality is probably a defect of lipid synthesis in the red cell stroma.

Haemoglobin is normally composed of a haem component and a protein moiety, globin. In normal adult haemoglobin (HbA) globin is composed of 4 peptide chains (2 α and 2 β), and in patients with abnormal haemoglobins (the *haemoglobinopathies*) there may be defects in the α or β chain structure (e.g. HbS) while in the second group the synthesis of β chains is suppressed (e.g. foetal Hb, HbF, and in HbA_2). In sickle cell anaemia and some other anaemias a variant form of Hb called HbS is produced due to a minor abnormality in the amino acid composition of the α or β chains of the globin molecule (e.g. the glutamic acid in peptide 4 of the β-chain is replaced by valine in HbS); HbS is less soluble than normal Hb, especially in the reduced state when it forms long chains which distort the red cells ("sickling phenomenon"). In thalassaemia misshapen cells are formed and there is a defect in adult haemoglobin production (synthesis of the β-chains of haemoglobin A is suppressed) and defective erythropoiesis and increased destruction both play a part in the anaemia of thalassaemia.

2. *Extrinsic (extracorpuscular) abnormality* due to development of an abnormal haemolytic mechanism.

In many forms globulins are produced which act as antibodies against the patient's own red cells (i.e. auto-antibodies)—*auto-immune acquired haemolytic anaemia*. This may be of unknown cause (idiopathic) in most adults, but in some is secondary to another disease (e.g. chronic lymphatic leukaemia, malignant lymphomas, various infections especially virus pneumonia, and disseminated lupus erythematosus). In addition drugs and chemicals and parasites may cause haemolytic anaemia, e.g.

the sulphones, lead poisoning;

malaria where there is destruction of red cells by the intracellular parasite with release of merozoites into the plasma;

occasionally due to primaquine, broad beans ("favism") where the idiosyncrasy is due to an inborn error of metabolism, namely a deficiency of the enzyme glucose-6-phosphate dehydrogenase (G-6PD) in the red cell (the enzyme catalyses glucose-6-phosphate $+$ NADP $\rightleftharpoons$ 6-phosphogluconate $+$ $NADPH_2$ and the $NADPH_2$ is used to produce reduced glutathione which is necessary for the maintenance of erythrocyte integrity).

Signs of Increased Red Cell Destruction

(a) Increased serum bilirubin—not an accurate measure of haemolysis for the level depends on the rate of red cell destruction and the rate of removal of the bilirubin from the plasma by the liver.

(b) Urobilinogen excretion—a group of faecal pigments which react with Ehrlich's aldehyde reagent: although faecal urobilinogen levels are not accurate indices of haemolysis, a proportion of the urobilinogen is normally absorbed and excreted in the urine (little in health, but increased urinary urobilinogen with haemolysis).

(c) Study of red cell survival—now usually done by "tagging" red cells with radioactive isotopes like ^{51}Cr: increased rate of fall of isotope level in the blood with increased haemolysis.

(d) Reduced plasma haptoglobulin levels—haemoglobin carried in plasma attached to plasma proteins called haptoglobulins: excess Hb from increased haemolysis causes a fall in plasma haptoglobulin levels.

(e) Compensating hyperplasia of the bone marrow may occur to counteract increased haemolysis—may cause skeletal or X-ray changes (e.g. in thalassaemia).

(f) Reticulocytosis—immature red cells in circulating blood: an attempt by the marrow to compensate for increased haemolysis.

Polycythaemia.—An increased number of red cells per unit volume of blood which may be due to:

I. a decrease in plasma volume due to loss of fluids in burns, persistent diarrhoea (e.g. cholera), etc.—*relative polycythaemia*;

II. an increase in the total number of red cells in the body:

(a) due to excess production of an erythropoietic factor *per se* e.g. kidney tumours and cysts, cerebellar haemangioblastoma (see Chapter II);

(b) due to a reduction of arterial blood oxygen content (probably with release of increased erythropoietic factor) e.g. cyanotic congenital heart disease, living at high altitudes;

(c) polycythaemia vera which is a progressive, ultimately fatal disease, with an excess production of all formed elements of the blood by a hyperplastic bone marrow. Like myeloid leukaemia, polycythaemia vera may terminate as myosclerosis (all included under the title "myeloproliferative disorders") in which there is a proliferative neoplasia of primitive mesenchymal tissue particularly in the bone marrow with interference with red cell production.

WHITE CELLS

The production of granulocytes appears to be stimulated by nucleoproteins and their derivatives from leucocytic nuclei. Leucocytes contain a large number of enzymes and are capable of digesting phagocytosed bacteria and cell debris and assist in the liquefaction of damaged tissues leading to pus formation. The alkaline phosphatase in neutrophils has been noted to be consistently low in chronic myelocytic leukaemia. In general the function of leucocytes is the defence of the body against infection and foreign substances; specific functions are:

neutrophil—phagocytosis of bacteria, especially pyogenic organisms;

eosinophil—transport of histamine in the blood; role uncertain but production stimulated by foreign proteins e.g. allergic disorders, parasite infestation;

basophil—carrier of histamine and heparin-like substance; role unclear;

lymphocyte—production and transport of antibody;

monocyte—phagocytosis of bacteria and cell debris.

Leucocyte counts are highest at birth (10 – 25,000 per cu.mm.) and fall to normal adult values of 4 – 10,000 per cu.mm. composed of:

neutrophils 40 – 75 per cent;

eosinophils 1 – 6 per cent;

basophils 1 per cent;

lymphocytes 20 – 50 per cent;

monocytes 2 – 10 per cent.

Leucocytosis.—An increase in circulating leucocytes either physiological (e.g. at birth) or pathological as below:

1. infection, especially with pyogenic cocci (staphylococcus, streptococcus, gonococcus, etc.) and pyogenic bacilli (*E. coli, Proteus, Ps. pyocyanea*) also in certain non-pyogenic infections (acute poliomyelitis, typhus, scarlet fever, rheumatic fever, etc.);

2. haemorrhage;
3. trauma e.g. operations, fractures, crush injuries, burns, myocardial infarction;
4. malignant disease especially with rapid growth and necrosis;
5. the myeloproliferative disorders of myeloid leukaemia and polycythaemia vera.

Lymphocytosis.—Infections which cause neutrophil leucocytosis in adults may cause increased lymphocyte levels in the blood in children e.g. pertussis. However lymphocytosis may be due to the exanthemata, lymphatic leukaemia, infectious mononucleosis.

Leucopenia.—May be defined as a reduction in the number of leucocytes below the normal lower limit (4000 per cu.mm.) and the causes are:

1. infections—viral, e.g. influenza, measles;
   rickettsia, e.g. typhus (mouse- or louse-borne);
   protozoa, e.g. malaria, kala-azar;
   bacteria, e.g. typhoid fever, brucellosis;
2. acute leukaemia;
3. drug induced (part of aplastic anaemia or else selective neutropoenia);
4. aplastic anaemia;
5. hypersplenism;
6. bone marrow infiltration (secondary carcinoma, malignant lymphomas, etc.);
7. idiopathic.

The usual cause of leucopenia is a fall in the number of circulating neutrophils.

Neutropenia (neutrophil count in blood below 2500/cu. mm.) and *agranulocytosis* (very few neutrophils in the peripheral blood + severe constitutional symptoms and ulcers).—The list of causes is as above for leucopenia, but there are only a few instances where neutropenia is severe enough to cause symptoms, e.g. acute leukaemia, idiopathic neutropenia and when induced by drugs. The drugs may cause an aplastic anaemia or else a selective neutropenia (the ones most likely to do this are amidopyrine and the thiouracil group of drugs). In amidopyrine sensitivity the drug combines with a body protein to form an antigenic complex which stimulates antibody production and finally agglutination of leucocytes with subsequent reduction in circulating neutrophils.

Eosinophilia.—Is present when the blood count exceeds 440/cu. mm. and may be due to allergic causes (asthma, drug allergy, serum sickness) or to parasites (filaria, trichinella, etc.).

Leukaemias.—Uncontrolled proliferation of leucocytic cells in the body due either to a virus infection or else of unknown aetiology. Damage to cells by ionising radiation can produce leukaemia (X-rays to patients with ankylosing spondylitis, increased incidence in American radiologists and survivors of the atomic bombs dropped on Japan), and a chromosomal abnormality leads to an increased incidence of leukaemia in Mongols (extra chromosome 21—see Chapter I).

Leukaemias are classified on the clinical course of the disease (acute, chronic) and the predominant cell present (myeloid, lymphatic, monocytic). Their clinical features are due to interference with red cell production and/or increased destruction, the defence of the body against infection and the infiltration of tissues with deposits of leukaemic cells.

RETICULO-ENDOTHELIAL SYSTEM

This is a tissue in the body with the common function of ingesting foreign particulate matter (i.e. the cells composing it are all macrophages), and was originally discovered by Aschoff from the capacity of the cells to remove colloid dyes of high molecular weight from the circulation. It is a physiological rather than an anatomical entity, e.g. Kupffer cells of the liver, splenic sinusoidal cells, histiocytes, circulating monocytes in the blood, lymphoid tissue (e.g. lymph nodes). Lymphoid tissue is composed of two types of cell, the lymphocyte and the reticulum cell.

Malignant lymphomas are diseases of the lymphatic system with progressive enlargement of tissue and multiplication of one or more of the cells present in lymph nodes:

1. tumours showing mainly lymphocytic proliferation, e.g. lymphosarcoma;
2. tumours showing mainly reticulum cell proliferation, e.g. reticulum cell sarcoma;
3. tumours showing mixed proliferation of both lymphocytes and reticulum cells, e.g. Hodgkin's disease (the commonest malignant lymphoma).

In addition there are a number of diseases in which the cells of the reticulo-endothelial system become filled with unusual substances, usually of a lipid nature (either secondary to a generalised disturbance of metabolism or else as a primary disorder of the reticulo-endothelial cells). The primary disorders include:

Niemann-Pick disease—accumulation of phospholipid;
Gaucher's disease—cerebrosides;
Schüller-Christian disease is now considered a proliferative disorder rather than a lipoidosis.

HAEMOSTASIS

There are three major components responsible for haemostasis:

vascular;
platelet;
coagulation;

and they act in a co-ordinated fashion to stop bleeding. Injury to a blood vessel starts the following train of events:

(a) reflex nervous vasoconstriction of the blood vessel;
(b) platelets adhere to the damaged edges of the vessel and to one another and eventually form an amorphous mass (viscous metamorphosis) with the liberation of serotonin which causes further vasoconstriction;
(c) the maintenance of haemostasis depends on the formation of a fibrin clot which later undergoes contraction and ultimately organisation.

Haemorrhagic disorders.—These may be due to vascular defects, platelet abnormalities or coagulation defects.

Vascular defects.—These are the commonest cause of bleeding disorders in clinical practice (causing petechiae or ecchymosis).

I. Congenital vascular defects, e.g. hereditary haemorrhagic telangiectasia.

II. Acquired vascular defects.

(a) Infections with toxic damage to blood vessels,
e.g. typhoid fever, subacute bacterial endocarditis with an allergic response to the infection;
e.g. scarlet fever, infectious mononucleosis;

(*b*) nutritional, e.g. scurvy due to deficient intake of vitamin C where there is defective formation of the intercellular cement substance of the capillary wall;

(*c*) metabolic disorders where there is some defect in the capillary endothelium, e.g. uraemia, Cushing's syndrome;

(*d*) hypersensitivity (to bacteria usually) with increased vascular permeability, e.g. anaphylactoid purpura;

(*e*) atrophy of collagen, e.g. senile purpura;

(*f*) idiopathic, e.g. simple easy bruising in women.

Platelet abnormalities.—Defect in the number of platelets usually (sometimes a qualitative defect). Platelets form a plug at the site of the vascular injury, release the vasoconstrictor serotonin, assist in blood coagulation (see later) and contain a retractile protein which is necessary for normal clot retraction (contracts under the influence of ATP). When the platelets are reduced in number below the lower normal limit of 150,000/cu. mm. the condition is called *thrombocytopenia.* Haemorrhage is common in thrombocytopenia and there is a positive tourniquet test, a prolonged bleeding time, impaired clot retraction but usually a normal coagulation time. Thrombocytopenia may be:

idiopathic—acute (especially in children) or the more common chronic form (usually adults) when it is secondary to:

(i) drugs which cause aplastic anaemia (e.g. gold, organic arsenicals, sulphonamides) or drugs which cause selective thrombocytopenia either due to a direct toxic effect on the bone marrow (e.g. salicylates) or a hypersensitivity reaction (e.g. Sedormid or quinidine where antibodies to a drug-platelet antigen are formed with subsequent destruction of platelets);

(ii) bone marrow infiltration, e.g. acute leukaemia, chronic lymphatic or myeloid leukaemia, secondary carcinoma, multiple myelomatosis, malignant lymphomas;

(iii) diminished bone marrow function, e.g. aplastic anaemia;

(iv) excessive destruction of platelets in the body, e.g. hypersplenism.

Coagulation defects.—The coagulation mechanism has two main functions:

   (i) To produce thrombin which helps platelets to make a platelet plug;

   (ii) to form a fibrin plug.

The mechanism of blood coagulation is as illustrated below, although there are numerous factors not indicated:

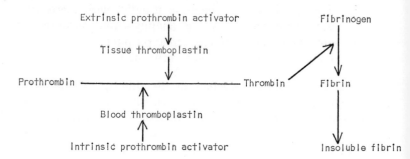

However, there are also mechanisms which help to maintain the fluidity of the blood within the vessels, the *fibrinolytic system* (see below).

There are several mechanisms available to preserve the fluidity of the blood:

   integrity of normal vascular endothelium;
   normal blood flow;
   presence of physiological anti-coagulants in the blood;
   physiological fibrinolysis.

Extrinsic prothrombin activator is formed by the interaction of tissue factors (which enter the blood from damaged cells) with calcium and the plasma clotting factors V, VII and X. Intrinsic prothrombin activator (or plasma thromboplastin) is formed when blood comes into contact with foreign surfaces and there is an activation of factors XI and XII causing an interaction with other clotting factors, especially factor VIII (anti-haemophiliac globulin, AHG), factor IX (Christmas factor), calcium, lipid from damaged platelets and factors X and V. Clinical disorders due to abnormalities in blood coagulation;

   (i) deficiency of coagulation factors, e.g.
      sex-linked recessive inheritance of factor VIII (AHG);
      deficiency as in haemophilia;

deficiency of factor IX (Christmas disease);

deficiency of AHG + a platelet abnormality (von Willebrand's disease; inherited as an autosomal dominant);

deficiency of factors VII, IX and X and prothrombin in vitamin K deficiency (vitamin K is necessary for their production); also due to anticoagulant therapy with coumarin or the indanedione group of drugs;

deficiency of fibrinogen (rarely congenital, usually acquired and often due to intravascular clotting with removal of fibrinogen as in incompatible blood transfusion, amniotic fluid embolism, concealed or accidental antepartum haemorrhage or intravascular tumour cell emboli: the defibrination syndrome).

(ii) Fibrinolysis.—This is the natural way in which formed fibrin is destroyed and blood clots are dissolved. The fibrinolytic mechanism is:

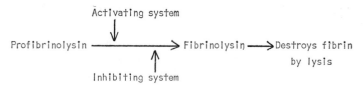

Activation of this system may occur with incompatible blood transfusions and amniotic fluid emboli, etc. (the acute defibrination syndrome) or leukaemia and disseminated prostatic carcinoma (chronic fibrinolysis). Streptokinase, isolated from filtrates of haemolytic streptococci, is a commercially available activator of this system. Epsilonaminocaproic acid will inhibit fibrinolysis.

(iii) Coagulation inhibitors may appear in the circulation and lead to a prolonged whole blood clotting time.

PLASMA

COMPOSITION 91 – 92 per cent water.

Proteins.

Inorganic constituents Na, Ca, K, Mg, P, I, Fe, etc.

Organic constituents—non-protein nitrogenous substances (urea, uric acid, creatinine, amino-acids) lipids (neutral fats phospholipids, cholesterol) glucose, antibodies, hormones, various enzymes (e.g. amylase, aspartate transaminase, etc.).

The normal plasma volume is about 5 per cent of body weight (i.e. approximately 3500 ml. for a 70 kg. man).

PLASMA PROTEINS

The total protein (6 – 7 G/100 ml. plasma) is composed of three fractions:

   (i) albumin;
   (ii) globulin;
   (iii) fibrinogen (0·3 – 0·4 G/100 ml. plasma).

These separate protein fractions can be separated by paper electrophoresis. Plasma or serum is placed on a piece of filter paper to which is added a buffer solution so that the proteins are ionised. When an electric field is applied across the filter paper the ionised proteins will move at a rate dependent on their net charge, mass and shape (the proteins on the paper strip are stained and the strip is then scanned by a densitometer and the pattern recorded on paper as illustrated. The size of the peaks represents the concentration of the specific protein fraction).

The normal concentrations are:

    G./100 ml.

albumin 3·6 – 5·2;
α globulin 0·5 – 1·2;
β globulin 0·5 – 1·2;
γ globulin 0·7 – 1·5.

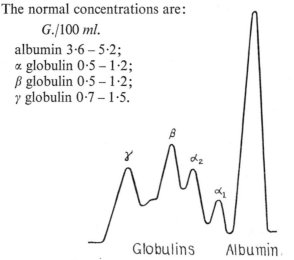

FIG. 6.—Paper electrophoretic pattern of plasma.

Factors Changing Plasma Protein Pattern

1. Infections—usually increased α-globulin in acute infections and γ-globulin in chronic ones. In some parasitic infections, e.g. kala-azar, there is a massive increase in γ-globulin.
2. Connective tissue disease—e.g. rheumatoid arthritis where there is a decrease in albumin with an increase in γ-globulin.
3. Malignant disease—no specific pattern except in multiple myelomatosis where there is a massive increase in γ-globulin.
4. Renal disease—when there is a large leak of albumin through the glomerular capillaries of the kidney, e.g. nephrotic syndrome, plasma albumin falls.
5. Auto-immune disease—there may be an increase in γ-globulin, e.g. Hashimoto's disease of the thyroid.
6. Hypoproteinaemia due to prolonged starvation, chronic liver disease (when albumin synthesis defective).

Sites of Production

(a) Albumin—the liver.
(b) Globulin—probably approx. 80 per cent from liver with rest mostly derived from the lymphocytes (some γ-globulin from plasma cells of the reticulo-endothelial system).
(c) Fibrinogen—liver.

Function

(i) Maintain osmotic pressure of plasma (see Starling's Law of capillaries in Chapter IV), mostly due to albumin which has the largest concentration of *particles* in the plasma.
(ii) Acid-base regulation by acting as buffers (constitute about one-sixth of buffering capacity of the blood).
(iii) Immunity.
(iv) Fibrinogen—for blood clotting mechanism.

Disorders of protein synthesis.—When these are primary disorders:

(a) Agammaglobulinaemia—serum γ-globulins greatly reduced:

    (i) congenital—familial, sex-linked recessive (males only);

    (ii) acquired—in leukaemias (deficient synthesis) and nephrosis (except loss).

In both there is increased susceptibility to infection.

(b) Paraproteinaemias. A given type (or clone) of stem cell of the reticulo-endothelial system develops along an abnormal line and produces an excess of a particular protein (such proteins are called paraproteins).

    (i) Myelomatosis in which an abnormal clone of plasma cells produce abnormal serum globulins, some of which may appear in the urine as Bence-Jones protein.

    (ii) Some cases of chronic lymphatic leukaemia and lymphosarcoma.

    (iii) Primary macroglobulinaemia (one type of large molecular weight globulin may precipitate on cooling—a *cryoglobulin*; may precipitate on adding the plasma to water in the water dilution test). Cryoglobulins may also occur in collagen diseases especially periarteritis nodosa, and also in myelomatosis. In the paraproteinaemias there is often a deficiency of normal antibody globulins and hence an increased tendency to infection.

(c) Afibrinogenaemia—may be acquired fibrinogen deficiency (e.g. from intravascular clotting or reduced formation) or congenital when it is a primary disorder of protein synthesis (autosomal recessive inheritance).

Immunoglobulins.—The immune globulins (or antibodies) move in the β or γ regions of paper electrophoresis and are composed as a pair of large polypeptide (heavy) chains each with a smaller piece (light chain) attached to it joined by -S-S-linkages. The chains are coils of amino-acids (molecular weight; light chains about 20,000, heavy chains about 55,000) and the immunoglobulins may be classified as follows:

I_gG—deals with bacterial infection (molecular weight about 150,000).

I_gA—secreted into saliva, gut and bronchial tree (probably protective action).

I$_g$M—macroglobulin (molecular weight about 1,000,000); similar type of globulin increased in Waldenstrom's macroglobulinaemia.

I$_g$D—action unknown.

I$_g$E—some connection with asthma.

In myelomatosis there is an homogeneous overproduction of globulins resembling I$_g$G or I$_g$A with only one (instead of two) light chains (because a neoplastic clone of myeloma cells has taken over production) and these have little or no functional capacity as antibodies.

Chapter VI

RESPIRATION

THE human body takes up oxygen from the air and by tissue metabolism produces carbon dioxide which has to be eliminated. The mechanisms concerned can be categorised as follows:

(a) Ventilation—the mechanical movement of gases in and out of the lungs.

(b) Distribution and diffusion—concerned with the movement of gases between alveolar gas and blood.

(c) Transport of gases by the blood.

(d) Tissue metabolism—considered extremely briefly in Chapter I (this is encompassed by the discipline, biochemistry).

VENTILATION

Lung volumes.—Gases are moved in and out of the lungs by muscle action and work is performed (the amount of work done depends on the resistance offered to movement by the lungs and chest cage). The volume of air inspired and subsequently expired is the *tidal volume* (approx. 500 ml. at rest), but about 150 ml. of this fills the air passages and does not come in contact with the alveoli (*dead space*); the remaining 350 ml. of air mixes with the air remaining in the lungs after a quiet expiration, the *functional residual capacity* (FRC approx. 2500 ml.).

At the end of a quiet expiration a further volume of gas can be expelled voluntarily (the expiratory reserve volume—ERC approx. 1200 ml.), but there remains gas in the lungs which cannot be expelled, the *residual volume* (RV approx. 1200 ml.) which is usually less than 30 per cent of the total lung capacity (of about 6000 ml.). The *vital capacity* is the volume of gas which can be expelled by a voluntary effort after a deep inspiration (VC approx. 5000 ml.). The various components of the vital capacity can be measured by a spirometer (a miniature gasholder), and the various lung volumes are summarised in the diagram below; measurement of residual volume requires a special technique.

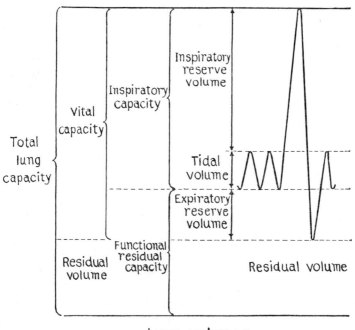

Lung volumes.

FIG. 7

Clinical application of respiratory function tests.—(The predicted normal for these tests for any individual is based on his age, surface area, etc.).

Vital capacity.—Serial changes may be a useful indication of progress in the course of a disease and 20 per cent below the predicted normal value is probably abnormal; a non-specific test really for many disorders will reduce the vital capacity, e.g.

reduction in functioning lung tissue, e.g. resection, collapse, pneumonia, fibrosis, congestion, tumour;

diminished ability of lungs to expand, e.g. pain, chest deformity, neuromuscular disease, pregnancy, effusion.

Forced expiratory volume in one second ($FEV_{1.0}$) is normally 80 per cent of vital capacity (another useful measure is the maximum mid-expiratory flow rate, MEF, which is the average rate of flow during the middle 50 per cent of FEV). Reduced in obstructive diseases, e.g. chronic bronchitis, asthma and emphysema (FEV may be below 40 per cent of VC in emphysema).

The *peak expiratory flow* (PEF) rate is easier to measure than the forced expiratory volume, using a Wright meter; after a maximum inspiration air is expelled as quickly as possible into the meter. Although the values obtained are rather variable, over 600 litres/min. in male is normal; serial measurements in asthma are a useful indication of the degree of bronchial spasm and the efficacy of bronchodilators; it is also reduced in emphysema and chronic bronchitis.

Maximum breathing capacity (MBC).—Total ventilation possible with maximum effort; measured for 15 secs. (to prevent unpleasant effects of prolonged hyperventilation) and expressed as litres/min. (in male about 150 litres/min. is normal).

Functional residual capacity (FRC) is one of the lung volumes which cannot be measured by spirometry and it has to be estimated indirectly;

open method—wash out all the nitrogen in the lungs with 100 per cent oxygen and measure the total amount of nitrogen evolved;

closed method—rebreathe from a bag containing 10 per cent helium until mixing is complete between the contents of the bag and the contents of the lungs (none is absorbed into the blood perfusing the lungs). Then measure the concentration of helium in bag (which is of known volume) and hence calculate the initial lung volume;

body plethysmography—subject enclosed in airtight box with mouth connected to a pressure transducer so that no air flow can occur; make an expiratory effort against this resistance when the gas in the lungs will be compressed and there will be a change in lung volume which is measured by the plethysmograph; from Boyle's law the volume of gas in the lungs can be calculated.

The FRC is increased in emphysema and asthma.

THE WORK OF BREATHING

| Work done ventilating the lungs (kg.m./min.) | = Force exerted by muscles of respir. | × Distance over which that force acts ($\equiv$ tidal volume × the frequency of breathing) |

Ventilatory work is done against the resistance of the chest wall, abdominal contents and lungs, and is partly:

(a) elastic—chief component of elastic resistance to inspiration is the recoil of the lung (especially due to surface tension effects in the alveoli);

(b) viscous or non-elastic—resistance to flow of air in the airways and resistance to movement of the tissues of lung and chest wall.

Elastic resistance.—The chief components of elastic resistance to inspiration are the true elastic tissue in the lung and surface tension effects. The recoil of the lungs provides the main force for expiration. The surface tension effects in the alveoli are due to the fluid which lines them, and surface tension forces tend to reduce their size. These effects are reduced by a surface-active lipoprotein (surfactant) lining the alveolar walls and preventing them sticking together. A deficiency of this lung surfactant is seen after cardiopulmonary by-pass, respiratory distress syndrome of the newborn, and also in emphysema. The elastic recoil of the lungs can be measured with an intra-oesophageal balloon attached to a pressure transducer (pressure in balloon = intrapleural pressure); the change in pressure produced by a volume change in the lung (measured with a special spirometer) is expressed as *compliance*.

$$\text{Compliance} = \frac{\text{change in lung volume (1.)}}{\text{change in intrapleural pressure (cm. water)}}$$

(Normal 0·2 litre/cm. H_2O).

The "stiffer" the lung, the less compliant it is.

Compliance is reduced by diffuse disorders of the lung, e.g. pulmonary fibrosis or congestion, respiratory disease of the newborn (due to abnormal surface tension forces), and disorders reducing volume change such as effusion or resection.

Non-elastic resistance.—Depends on the movement of air and tissues, and is subdivided into two components:

(i) resistance to flow of air in the airways—depends on airway diameter, also the density and viscosity of gas and amount of turbulence, e.g. breathing 20 per cent oxygen in helium which is less dense than air, reduces the work of breathing; increased airway resistance in emphysema, asthma, bronchitis;

(ii) resistance to movement of the tissues of the lung and chest wall; in normal breathing this contributes about a third of total non-elastic resistance.

The work of breathing is done against (a) elastic and (b) non-elastic loads, and if compliance is reduced (e.g. pneumonia, pulmonary fibrosis, pulmonary congestion) a higher breathing rate is advantageous, whereas with increased airway resistance (e.g. asthma, bronchitis) an increased depth of breathing is better. Normally the work of breathing is about 0·3 kg.m./min. at rest, but in mitral stenosis (where there is pulmonary congestion) and emphysema this may increase tenfold, and this extra work requires oxygen (usually the oxygen cost of breathing is about 1 – 3 per cent of the total body oxygen consumption but in emphysema this may rise to 20 per cent, and on exercise this proportion rises rapidly).

Dyspnoea is an unpleasant awareness of respiratory effort, and usually increased work of breathing relative to ventilation causes it (although this does not account for the dyspnoea of disordered neuromuscular function, e.g. poliomyelitis, which may be also due to nervous reflexes from receptors within the chest wall when the distension of the chest is reduced). Hence any disorder increasing the work of breathing can cause dyspnoea.

Hypoventilation.—A list of the causes will be put here for convenience although a full understanding of the mechanisms involved will depend on information later in the chapter:

1. depression of the respiratory centre, e.g. morphine;
2. interference with neuromuscular function, e.g. curare, poliomyelitis, myasthenia gravis;
3. diseases of the respiratory muscles;
4. limitation of movement of the thorax;
5. limitation of movement of the lungs;
6. pulmonary diseases, e.g. atelectasis, pneumonia, obstructive lesions of the upper and lower respiratory tracts.

Hypoventilation has an effect on blood gases causing:

hypoxaemia (arterial P_{O_2} reduced; normal 104 mm.Hg);

carbon dioxide retention (increased arterial P_{CO_2}; normal 40 mm.Hg);

respiratory acidosis (see Chapter IV).

UTILISATION OF VENTILATION

Air has to come into contact with blood in the alveolar wall for adequate gas exchange and the factors involved will be considered below under (a) uniformity of ventilation, (b) ratio of ventilation to perfusion of the lung area with blood (ventilation-perfusion ratio).

(a) Uniformity of Ventilation

Normally there are regional differences in the ventilation of the lung which depend on posture, depth of ventilation and exercise, e.g. in the erect posture ventilation per unit volume of lung in man is greater at the bases than the apices. Distortion of the bronchial tree and destruction of lung tissue by disease cause greater maldistribution of inspired air. The mixing efficiency of the lungs can be measured by studying the fall in concentration of nitrogen in end-expired air while breathing pure oxygen (using a nitrogen analyser); in normal person, after 7 mins. breathing, conc. less than 2·5 per cent nitrogen, but if the gas distribution is not uniform this percentage is increased; measuring the fall in helium concentration when rebreathed from a closed spirometer (using a helium meter).

(b) Ventilation-perfusion Ratio

Ventilation-perfusion abnormalities are the commonest cause of hypoxia and hypercapnia in clinical medicine; in the bronchitic and asthmatic patient hypoxaemia is mainly due to profound ventilation-perfusion imbalance in the lung and alveolar hypoventilation is not usually an important factor in the development of arterial desaturation in these disorders. In normal subjects there are regional differences in ventilation (see (a) above) and also in blood flow, e.g. in the erect subject ventilation is reduced at the apex and also blood flow in comparison with the base (blood flow reduced more than ventilation so some ventilated lung at the apex is not perfused with blood). Parts of the lung with high blood flow in relation to ventilation act as a shunt for blood, i.e. by-pass aerated lung, and this can cause oxygen desaturation of arterial blood. The perfusion of under-ventilated area of lung can be estimated from the difference in oxygen tension between alveolar gas and arterial blood ($PA_{O_2} - Pa_{O_2}$ difference; normally 9 mm.Hg). Mechanisms responsible for the normal fine adjustment of blood flow to ventilation are not clear but hypoxia is one (causes local reduction in pulmonary blood flow by vasoconstriction—see Chapter III). When blood flow and ventilation are not matched there is impaired gas exchange in the lung, e.g. emphysema, pneumonia, collapse, pulmonary infarction; this leads mainly to reduced oxygen tension rather than increased carbon dioxide tension. Cyanosis at rest without an anatomical shunt is usually due to perfusion of under-ventilated lung (if the patient breathes pure oxygen there will be no increase in arterial oxygen tension if anatomical shunt but there will be an increase in arterial oxygen tension if there is a pulmonary cause for the initial arterial desaturation).

Diffusion

The gas in the alveoli and in the blood has to be exchanged across the wall of the alveolus by the process of diffusion (gas molecules pass from region of high partial pressure to one lower). The volume of gas transferred in unit time (D_L) depends on the surface area of the alveoli and the thickness of the membrane through which the gas has to diffuse (essentially the alveolar wall and lining fluid).

Diffusion of carbon dioxide is never limited by disturbances in diffusion although oxygen movement may be for it is much slower. Diffusion rate is measured in man using carbon monoxide (D_{LCO}) and it may be changed in diseases causing thickening of the alveolar wall—the *alveolar-capillary block syndrome* which may be produced by sarcoidosis, berylliosis, asbestosis, scleroderma, lymphangitis carcinomatosa, diffuse interstitial pulmonary fibrosis. Impaired gas diffusion due to the above will usually only produce cyanosis on exercise (however, it is now thought that thickening of the membrane could not interfere with oxygen exchange to a sufficient degree to produce cyanosis, but that the cause of the low D_L is really interference with ventilation-perfusion relationships).

NEURAL AND CHEMICAL CONTROL OF VENTILATION

Peripheral Neural Mechanisms

Efferent nerves.—The phrenic nerves innervate the diaphragm, and intercostal nerves supply the intercostal muscles and T7 – L1 nerves the abdominal muscles. Inspiration is produced by centrally co-ordinated contraction of the inspiratory muscles; inspiration grows to a peak and is then abruptly terminated.

Afferent discharge which is effective in controlling and modifying ventilation may be carried in:

glossopharyn-⎤ impulses from carotid and aortic bodies
geal nerve (IX) ⎬ which contain chemoreceptors responding
vagus (X) ⎦ to changes in blood gas tensions;

vagus (X) impulses from stretch receptors in the lungs (basis of Hering-Breuer reflex—inflation of the lungs tends to terminate inspiration, collapse of the lungs initiates inspiration);

various somatic nerves—noxious impulses from various parts of the body, e.g. gasp (inspiration) when cold shower turned on;

various proprioceptive nerves—from proprioceptor organs of limbs (and possibly other muscles) which are of prime importance in explaining the hyperventilation of exercise.

Cough.—Results from mechanical or chemical irritation of endings in the respiratory passages while sneeze is due to irritation of the nasal mucosa (supplied by trigeminal nerve V). Both cough and sneeze are reflex phenomena.

Central Neural Mechanisms

Cerebral cortex.—Respiration is subject to voluntary control, but possibly the limbic system is also involved (breathing is, of course, a component of emotional expression—see Chapter X).

Pons and medulla.—Electrical stimulation of specific areas can cause inspiratory apnoea (apneusis), change in rate, etc., and these respiratory centres can be defined in the following manner:

 (i) pneumotaxic centre—situated high in the pons; if removed with vagi cut then prolonged inspiration or apneusis;

 (ii) apneustic centre—a pontine area below the pneumotaxic centre which produces the apneusis mentioned above (i.e. when pneumotaxic centre and vagi removed).

 (iii) medullary respiratory centre—lies in the reticular substance of the medulla and contains two ill-defined centres, an inspiratory and an expiratory centre, which are connected such that the activity of one tends to inhibit the activity of the other (although the inspiratory centre is dominant).

Although (i) and (ii) probably exist their role is normally probably unimportant, and the important central controller of ventilation is the medullary respiratory centre.

The respiratory centres maintain rhythmic ventilatory activity but the proprioceptive impulses (Hering-Breuer reflex) determine the characteristics of amplitude and frequency of respiration (cut the vagi and the respiratory rate becomes slower and deeper due to removal of the Hering-Breuer reflex).

Chemical Control of Ventilation

Hypoxia (decreased P_{O_2}), changes in carbon dioxide tension and H^+ ion concentration in the blood also alter ventilation. The carotid body (which lies just above the carotid sinus) and aortic body respond to change in arterial P_{O_2} rather than oxygen content, and impulses pass up IX and X nerves respectively to the medullary respiratory centres. In the presence of reduced arterial P_{O_2} these chemoreceptors also respond to changes in blood P_{CO_2} and pH. However, increased arterial carbon dioxide tension still increases ventilation after denervation of the peripheral chemoreceptors and this is due to a central effect (a direct one on the medullary respiratory centres).

Hypoxia stimulates ventilation *solely* by its effect on the carotid and aortic chemoreceptors (when these are denervated hypoxia actually reduces, not stimulates, ventilation by a central depressant action on the respiratory centres). These receptors do contribute to the ventilatory drive in man at sea level (a sudden change in inspired gas from air to pure oxygen in man produces a fall in ventilation). The effects of hypoxia and increased carbon dioxide tension in blood are greater than the additive effects of each (i.e. there is potentiation of these two stimuli with regard to ventilation).

Carbon dioxide can act on the respiratory centres directly and indirectly (through the carotid and aortic chemoreceptors as shown originally by Heymans). It is probable that in normo-capnia the reflexogenic response to carbon dioxide stimulus is only minor, but in severe hypercapnia when the respiratory centres respond poorly to the direct carbon dioxide stimulus, the reflex pathway assumes greater importance. Even the reduction in arterial P_{CO_2} associated with a sigh can produce measurable hypoventilation in man showing that changes in carbon dioxide tension constitute a normal physiological system for ventilatory control.

H+ ion—In prolonged metabolic acidosis, e.g. diabetic acidosis, metabolic carbon dioxide production is unchanged so that hyperventilation must be due to increased H^+ ion concentration in blood for there is a fall in blood P_{CO_2}; in fact if there were no hypocapnia, the hyperventilation due to acidosis would be much greater. In contrast large doses of bicarbonate produce metabolic alkalosis with an increase in pH (i.e. fall in blood concentration of H^+ ion) and an increase in P_{CO_2} (which normally causes hyperventilation) yet there is decreased ventilatory activity. Hence carbon dioxide and H^+ ion are ventilatory stimuli, and they are related biochemically through the Henderson-Hasselbalch equation (see Chapter IV).

Other Factors Regulating Ventilation

(*a*) Increase in arterial blood pressure can produce hypoventilation (and hypotension can produce hyperventilation) by affecting either the carotid and aortic pressoreceptors or chemoreceptors in animal experiments (normal role of these baroreceptors in ventilatory control in man is not clear).

(*b*) Cerebral influences can change ventilation, e.g. voluntary hyperventilation.

(*c*) Proprioceptive receptors—passive movements of the limbs causes hyperventilation in man (and this effect is abolished by a spinal block with local anaesthetic). In animals stimulation of nerve fibres to muscle spindles will produce reflex hyperventilation.

(*d*) Intense stimulation of sense organs in the skin, e.g. excitation of pain receptors causing hyperventilation (also sneeze and cough reflexes are changes in ventilation due to sense organ stimulation in nose and tracheobronchial tree).

(*e*) Pulmonary mechanoreceptors—stretch receptors in the walls of the terminal bronchioles and their ramifications (the Hering-Breuer reflex—see above).

Regulation of ventilation at rest.—There is an oxygen stimulus (accounts for about 10 – 15 per cent of observed ventilation), carbon dioxide and H^+ ion stimuli to which the respiratory centres are very sensitive; the role of other factors at rest is not clear.

Regulation of ventilation during muscular exercise.—The instantaneous increase in ventilation is due to neurogenic stimuli (either proprioceptive from the muscles and joints or cerebral in origin), then after about 15 seconds humoral stimuli also take part (carbon dioxide and H^+ ion stimuli, and during severe exercise increased ventilation can be caused by increased level of circulating adrenaline). The role of the baroreceptors, is not clear but increase in the temperature of blood perfusing the brain (i.e. central hyperthermia) is probably not a stimulus in man (although a strong stimulus to tachypnoea in the dog).

GAS TRANSPORT

Oxygen and carbon dioxide are present in the blood in two forms, dissolved and chemically combined.

Dissolved oxygen.—At sea level, breathing room air, the

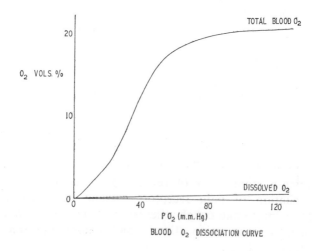

BLOOD O_2 DISSOCIATION CURVE

partial pressure of oxygen in arterial blood, Pa_{O_2}, is about 95 mm.Hg, and according to Henry's law the amount of dissolved oxygen in this arterial blood is 0·29 ml./100 ml. blood

(0·29 vols. per cent). In venous blood Pv_{O_2} = 40 mm.Hg and dissolved oxygen is 0·12 vols. per cent. When breathing 100 per cent oxygen, Pa_{O_2} may reach 640 mm.Hg and dissolved oxygen about 2 vols. per cent.

Chemically bound oxygen.—The blood oxygen content of arterial blood is about 20 vols. per cent (0·3 vols. per cent dissolved, the rest combined with haemoglobin). There is a relationship between the oxygen content of blood and the partial pressure of oxygen to which it is exposed, and this can be expressed in graphical form as the blood oxygen dissociation curve. An increase in temperature displaces the curve to the right (at same P_{O_2}, the higher the temperature the lower will be the oxygen content of the blood). Also the P_{CO_2} to which the blood is exposed alters the curve, displacing it to the right as the P_{CO_2} is increased (*the Bohr effect*). Both these features assist displacement of oxygen from blood at the tissue level (where the temperature and P_{CO_2} are higher).

Haemoglobin (see Chapter V) contains 0·33 per cent by weight of iron and when combined with oxygen (oxyHb) is red while the non-oxygenated state is purple. A gram of haemoglobin can bind 1·34 ml. oxygen. If exposed to carbon monoxide, carboxyHb is formed and will not release oxygen to the tissues (the affinity of Hb for CO is 200 – 300 times greater than its affinity for oxygen).

Dissolved carbon dioxide.—Dissolved carbon dioxide is found in plasma and red cells. In arterial blood there are 2·7 vols. per cent dissolved carbon dioxide at a pressure of 41 mm.Hg, and in venous blood 3·07 vols. per cent.

Combined carbon dioxide.—Carbon dioxide entering red cells combines with water to produce bicarbonate ions (under the influence of the enzyme, carbonic anhydrase) which combine with K^+ ions inside the red cell. Part of the bicarbonate ion formed inside the red cell diffuses into the plasma while chloride ions diffuse from plasma into the red cell (the *Hamburger interchange* or chloride shift). Carbon dioxide is also combined with the globin part of haemoglobin yielding carbaminohaemoglobin ($HbCO_2$). Hence red cells and haemoglobin play a considerable role in the transport of carbon dioxide in blood, even though most of the carbon dioxide is found in the plasma as bicarbonate ion.

Carbon dioxide carriage in vols. per cent:

	Arterial Blood	Venous Blood
dissolved	2·7	3·1
bicarbonate ion	43·9	47·0
carbaminohaemoglobin	2·4	3·9
total	49·0	54·0
P_{CO_2} (mm.Hg)	41	47·5

The relationship between blood carbon dioxide and the partial pressure of CO_2 to which it is exposed are graphically shown by the blood carbon dioxide dissociation curve. At any CO_2 partial pressure, the CO_2 content of blood decreases when the

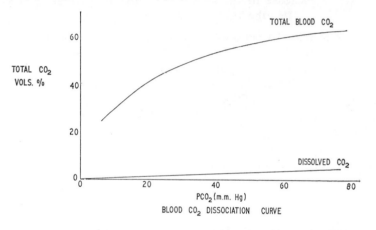

BLOOD CO_2 DISSOCIATION CURVE

partial pressure of oxygen increases (the *Haldane effect*), and this helps the blood take up carbon dioxide from the tissues and unload carbon dioxide at the alveoli.

Cyanosis

A purplish colour of the skin, nail-beds and mucosae which occurs when capillary blood contains more than 5 G. non-oxygenated haemoglobin per 100 ml. blood. The causes are:

(i) anatomical right to left shunt (very little rise in per cent oxygen saturation of blood when breathing 100 per cent oxygen);

(ii) pulmonary causes—rise in blood oxygen saturation on breathing 100 per cent oxygen. The commonest pulmonary cause is maldistribution of ventilation and blood flow which causes cyanosis at rest (diffusion defects usually cause cyanosis only on exercise);

(iii) stasis-reduced blood flow, e.g. cold weather, peripheral circulatory failure, etc.

Hypoxia

The tissues lack oxygen, and the causes were originally classified by Barcroft in the following simple manner:

anoxic—lack of oxygen in the inspired air;

anaemic—reduced capacity of the blood to carry oxygen;

stagnant—reduced blood flow to tissues;

histotoxic—inability of the tissues to utilise oxygen (e.g. cytochrome system poisoned by cyanide).

The following is a more up-to-date classification where hypoxia may be due to:

1. decrease of partial pressure of oxygen in inspired air, e.g. at high altitudes;

2. decrease of partial pressure of oxygen in the alveolar air consequent on alveolar hypoventilation, e.g. paralysis of respiratory muscles, abnormalities of the ventilatory apparatus (pulmonary fibrosis, rigid or deformed chest); note that alveolar hypoventilation causes hypoxia $+$ hypercapnia (i.e. asphyxia);

3. marked unevenness of ventilation/perfusion ratios, e.g. pulmonary emphysema;

4. decrease in oxygen diffusing capacity of the lung (alveolar-capillary block), e.g. the pulmonary granulomatoses (see above); note that the arterial P_{CO_2} is not increased because carbon dioxide diffuses much more rapidly than O_2;

5. an abnormally high venous flow into arterialised blood returning from the lungs, e.g. congenital heart disease with right-to-left shunt (Fallot's tetralogy, pulmonary hypertensive patent ductus arteriosus).

In the above 1 – 4 there is decreased arterial P_{O_2} and oxygen saturation covered by Barcroft's "anoxic anoxia".

6. decrease in concentration of functional haemoglobin, e.g. any anaemia, presence of carboxyhaemoglobin in the blood;

7. insufficient amount of oxygen supplied to the tissues because of reduced blood flow (ischaemic hypoxia—equivalent to stagnant hypoxia of Barcroft), e.g. vascular occlusion, vasomotor disturbances (e.g. Raynaud's disease and syndrome), reduced cardiac output;

8. poisoning of enzyme systems used in cell respiration.

The term "hypoxia" is correct but "anoxia" is freely substituted, for to be pedantic is to deny the use of the word "anaemia".

Respiratory failure can be defined biochemically as an arterial oxygen tension below 60 mm.Hg or an arterial carbon dioxide tension above 49 mm.Hg due to respiratory disease. Clinically the commonest cause is failure of satisfactory ventilation (although a high arterial P_{CO_2} can occur in metabolic alkalosis and a low P_{O_2} in right-to-left shunts which by-pass the lungs, these do not constitute respiratory failure). It can be divided into acute and chronic forms:

Acute respiratory failure occurs in acute laryngeal oedema, severe asthma and bronchitis; barbiturate overdosage; it should be treated by counteracting the primary cause (e.g. adrenaline for first, bronchodilators like isoprenaline, and steroids for severe asthma; chemotherapy for acute bronchitis) while also clearing the airway (check position of tongue, suction, endotracheal tube), and, if not sufficient, assist ventilation (e.g. intermittent positive pressure respirator), while increasing the oxygen content of the inspired air can be employed if ventilation with room air is inadequate. With carbon monoxide poisoning ventilation with high pressure oxygen is very effective.

Chronic respiratory failure—usually due to bronchitis, often with emphysema.

There are two types of respiratory failure delineated biochemically:

(i) Low Pa_{O_2} with normal or low Pa_{CO_2}—disorders of diffusion or distribution of ventilation and blood flow, e.g. alveolar-capillary block, pneumonia, massive collapse of the lung, and here oxygen therapy is of great help.

(ii) Low Pa_{O_2} with raised Pa_{CO_2}—due to alveolar hypoventilation (causes as given previously). Note that a Pa_{CO_2} above 100 mm.Hg may produce narcosis.

Chapter VII

THE GASTRO-INTESTINAL TRACT

Saliva.—The salivary glands secrete saliva which contains the enzyme amylase (a protein of molecular weight about 50,000 containing calcium which splits starch and glycogen into maltose) and the secretory activity is regulated mainly by parasympathetic nerves:

stimulate parasympathetic nerves→flow of saliva + vasodilatation of gland
ditto + atropine →flow of saliva reduced but
no effect on the vaso-
dilatation

It is now considered that the vasodilatation is due to the inter-action of plasma with an enzyme released by the activity of nerve endings which produces an atropine-resistant vaso-dilator, bradykinin.

Deficiency of saliva causes dry mouth (xerostomia), e.g. dehydration; Sjögren's syndrome where there is destruction of the salivary glands (due to rheumatoid arthritis and other collagen diseases); atropine which blocks the action of para-sympathetic nerves on the glands.

Swallowing.—There are three stages:

Oral phase—after mastication the bolus of food is forced into the pharynx by movements of the tongue; this is a voluntary act, whereas the next two stages are involuntary (controlled by swallowing centres in medulla); the impact of the bolus of food against the pharynx is the stimulus that sets off the reflex movements of swallowing.

The pharyngeal stage—the soft palate blocks off the naso-pharynx, the larynx is pulled up and food passes on either side of the epiglottis or over it (after the entrance to larynx closed by the action of the pharyngeal constrictors on the epiglottis).

Oesophageal stage—food falls under the influence of gravity followed by peristaltic waves in the oesophagus (i.e. food falls as the oesophagus relaxes rather than being propelled by a forceful peristaltic wave). The lower end of the oesophagus relaxes reflexly shortly after swallowing begins.

Dysphagia—pain or difficulty in swallowing.

(a) During mastication with any painful lesion of the mouth, e.g. dental abscess, oral ulcers; carcinoma of the tongue may interfere with the mobility of the tongue; painful lesions in the throat (e.g. tonsillitis, infectious mononucleosis) will also interfere with swallowing.

(b) Painless causes of dysphagia are those associated with neuromuscular disturbances to deglutition, especially lesions of the motor nuclei of the lower cranial nerves (e.g. bulbar poliomyelitis, syringobulbia, motor neurone disease, diphtheria) and lesions at the neuromuscular junction (e.g. myasthenia gravis).

Obstructive lesions may cause dysphagia (e.g. carcinoma of the thyroid, secondary deposits in the cervical lymph glands, pharyngeal diverticulum) and atrophic changes in pharynx cause dysphagia in iron-deficiency anaemia (Plummer-Vinson syndrome).

(c) The most important cause of dysphagia in the third stage of swallowing is carcinoma of the oesophagus; some other causes are strictures, and achalasia of the cardia. In achalasia the lower end of the oesophagus does not relax in a co-ordinated manner in response to the initiation of swallowing and there is a disorganisation of the normal peristaltic waves in the body of the oesophagus (this causes a physiological block); a similar picture occurs when the ganglion cells of the oesophagus are destroyed (e.g. by the parasite *Trypanosoma cruzi*) or the wall is infiltrated (scleroderma) and peristaltic waves are abnormal.

For control of *gastro-oesophageal reflux* there must be a length of intra-abdominal oesophagus together with a pressure barrier at the gastro-oesophageal junction (e.g. in hiatus hernia where the sphincter is displaced into the thorax, reflux can occur even when there is a good lower oesophageal sphincter barrier). In addition the angle at which the oesophagus enters the stomach and possibly a pinching effect near the diaphragm (due to the difference between negative intrathoracic and positive intra-abdominal pressures) help to prevent reflux into the oesophagus. Irritating fluid entering the oesophagus due to gastro-oesophageal reflux causes retrosternal discomfort ("heartburn"). Most common cause of reflux is a sliding hiatus hernia which removes two of the four possible preventive mechanisms.

GASTRIC FUNCTION

The stomach has two functions, secretory and mechanical.
Gastric secretion.—Most of the gastric secretion comes from the gastric glands and it contains:

mucigen—from surface cells; contains various mucoproteins which protect against mechanical and chemical injury to the mucosa; in addition blood group substances may be secreted in gastric mucus; Castle's intrinsic factor is probably a fraction of gastric mucoprotein (essential for effective absorption of vitamin B_{12} from the small intestine; deficiency due to gastric atrophy causes Addisonian anaemia—see Chapter V). There is a correlation between Group O (i.e. no blood group antigens of ABO series—see Chapter V) and duodenal ulcer, possibly because of deficient protection of the duodenal mucosa from trauma;
pepsinogen—released in response to vagal stimulation from chief cells (with molecular weight of 42,500 and composed of pepsin and peptide fragments) and becomes pepsin under influence of acid;
hydrochloric acid—from parietal cells (none in the pylorus) at a concentration of 160 mEq./litre which cannot be increased although there can be excessive production of HCl per unit time. There is a gross excess of HCl produced in the Zollinger-Ellison syndrome.

The hormone *gastrin* (a 17-amino-acid polypeptide) stimulates the secretion of both hydrochloric acid and pepsin by the stomach (exists in two forms, gastrin I without sulphate and gastrin II with an ethereal sulphate); an analogue of the C-terminal tetrapeptide amide called pentagastrin has been made and is used in man to test gastric secretory capacity (the pentagastrin test, using $6\mu g./Kg.$ subcutaneously, has now superseded the augmented histamine test as a measure of *parietal cell mass*). The role of histamine in gastric secretion has still not been settled but there is doubt regarding any function for it in man. The vagus stimulates the parietal cells and also causes the release of gastrin into the circulation: it has been suggested that gastrin may in fact be a transmitter substance like acetylcholine. When a meal is eaten there are three phases in the secretion of gastric juices:

> *Cephalic phase*—secretion caused by vagus only (remember Pavlov's sham feeding experiments) which excites secretion of acid by stomach by direct cholinergic stimulation of the oxyntic glands and cholinergic stimulation of release of gastrin from the pyloric glands.

> *Gastric phase*—mechanical distension ⎫ — gastrin (hormone)
> protein products in the stomach ⎬ liberated in antrum
> vagal stimulation ⎭
>
> fundus glands secrete acid and water (not pepsin)—some acid released by *direct* vagal action on oxyntic cells.

(In the Zollinger-Ellison syndrome non-insulin-secreting pancreatic adenoma produce a material now considered identical with the antral hormone, gastrin).

> Acid in antrum—inhibition of gastrin release (i.e. a self-regulating secretory system): mechanism involved is unknown.

> *Intestinal phase*—excited by the presence of food in intestine—
> hormone release
> (? gastrin)
> |
> gastric secretion

The amount of digestion undertaken by the stomach is small, but its mechanical or "hopper" function is important. The best test of gastric secretion used to be the augmented histamine test (now superseded by pentagastrin test), but this is not of much value in the diagnosis of peptic ulcers, etc. (although used to assess peptic ulcers), but only for achlorhydria (as in Addisonian anaemia) and the Zollinger-Ellison syndrome where there is a very high resting acid secretion compared with that seen with histamine stimulation (can test for HCl secretion by the stomach using a cation-exchange resin + attached blue dye—"Diagnex blue"—the dye is detached in the presence of H^+ ions and excreted in the urine; this test is now outmoded for it gives many false results). Insulin is now commonly used to estimate vagal action on the stomach; probably acts to stimulate gastric secretion due to hypoglycaemic stress on the hypothalamus.

An erosion of the mucosa, i.e. an ulcer, can occur in any part of the gastro-intestinal tract exposed to gastric juice, e.g.

stomach;
first part of duodenum;
lower end of oesophagus;
areas where abnormal presence of gastric mucosa, e.g. Meckel's diverticulum.

Although these are all mucosal erosions the mechanisms responsible are different and they are not an homogenous group. These ulcers give rise to certain symptoms related to food intake, especially pain which is only partly due to the direct contact of HCl with the ulcer. It is following surgical treatment of these ulcers in the stomach and duodenum that the "hopper" function of the stomach is affected (see Gastric motility). Vagotomy is used extensively in the surgical treatment of peptic ulcer and it has been shown in man to reduce the basal secretion of acid and to abolish the response to cephalic vagal stimulants such as insulin hypoglycaemia. There are a variety of disorders which can follow stomach resection in man ranging from the common distended bloated feeling to negative nitrogen balance and weight loss.

Gastric motility.—There is little muscular activity of the stomach in the resting state but when food enters the stomach it relaxes to accommodate it without a change in intragastric pressure. Gastric peristaltic waves mix the food with the gastric secretions and the stomach empties by distal relaxation of muscle sphincters rather than forceful peristalsis (emptying stops mainly due to active constriction of the pyloric ring). Gastric emptying is delayed by emotional distress, haemorrhage and the composition of the food (e.g. fats, hypertonic glucose). It is possible to assess gastric motility clinically by looking for visible peristalsis, e.g. readily seen in congenital pyloric stenosis. The stomach is an important container for food, releasing it for digestion gradually. When this "hopper" function is interfered with then secondary small intestinal disturbances occur.

After gastric surgery the ability of the stomach to hold food is changed sometimes and this may cause:

1. The dumping syndrome—epigastric distension and nausea, often with vasomotor changes (e.g. sweating, tachycardia) due to distension of jejunum with hypertonic solutions after gastric resection.
2. Hypoglycaemic attacks due to rapid emptying of stomach after operation with consequent rapid absorption of sugar and excessive insulin secretion causing hypoglycaemia about three hours after a meal.
3. Anaemia—usually of the iron-deficiency type due to impaired iron absorption; occasionally megaloblastic anaemia occurs due to impaired vitamin B_{12} absorption.
4. Diarrhoea—due to rapid transit of food through the intestine.
5. Malabsorption—steatorrhoea and abnormal calcium absorption can occur.
6. The by-passed (afferent) piece of small intestine may not empty properly causing vomiting (the afferent loop syndrome).

All these are due to a change in the "hopper" function of the stomach. The duodenum can inhibit gastric emptying by releasing a hormone, *enterogastrone*, when emulsified fat and hypertonic solutions of sugars and peptone come in contact with the duodenal mucosa (possibly osmoreceptors in the duodenum are involved).

SMALL INTESTINAL FUNCTION: DIGESTION AND ABSORPTION

Digestion.—Due to enzymes in:

(i) the pancreatic juice (the exocrine function of the pancreas; the endocrine function is production of insulin and glucagon—see Chapter II);
proteases, e.g. trypsinogen, chymotrypsinogen, etc. (all split proteins to polypeptides and then to amino-acids);
amylase (glycogen and starch split to maltose);
maltase (maltose to glucose);
lipase (fats to tri-, di- and monoglycerides, and fatty acids and glycerol);

(ii) the intestinal juice (succus entericus) secreted by the glands of the small intestine;
enterokinase (converts trypsinogen to trypsin);

peptidases, amylase, lactase, maltase, invertase, lipase, mucinase.

Secretion occurs spontaneously but can be excited by various substances locally (no effect from vagus) and also there is an unknown humoral mechanism affecting secretion (not secretin or gastrin).

The enzymes are probably intracellular (i.e. not found in centrifuged succus entericus). There is a rapid turnover of intestinal mucosal cells reflected in the high mitotic rate (hence radiosensitivity and the gastro-intestinal signs of overdosage of ionising radiations—see Chapter I).

The commonest movements of the small gut are irregular segmenting contractions which may be stationary or propagated for some distance down the intestine; they have a propulsive function if there is a gradient of pressure on the two sides of the contraction. Intestinal movements are modified by external nervous stimuli, stimuli from the gut lumen, environmental factors (e.g. gut atony in hypokalaemia, increased transit rate with thyrotoxicosis, diarrhoea in the carcinoid syndrome, etc.).

Control of pancreatic secretion.—Although parasympathetic stimulation increases pancreatic secretion, nervous influences (secretory nerves are all cholinergic) play a minor part in the regulation of its secretion (the cephalic stage of pancreatic secretion) which is essentially under the control of humoral materials. However vagal action on the gland together with vagal release of gastrin prepares the gland for the stimulus of these humoral agents.

Secretin (a 27-amino-acid polypeptide hormone produced when acid, peptones or *hypo*tonic solutions come in contact with duodenum)—stimulates secretion of bicarbonate by pancreas;

pancreozymin (hormone produced by small intestinal mucosa when foodstuffs come in contact with it; causes increased secretion of pancreatic enzymes): cholecystokinin is probably identical with pancreozymin;

gastrin also stimulates the secretion of pancreatic juice, bicarbonate and enzymes.

The principal diseases of the pancreas are cystic fibrosis (mucoviscidosis), acute, relapsing and chronic pancreatitis, tumours and kwashiorkor (causing atrophy and fibrosis of pancreas).

DISORDERS OF SMALL INTESTINAL SECRETION

1. Genetic deficiency of disaccharides of the *succus entericus* causing a specific intolerance to certain sugars and hence diarrhoea, e.g. lactase deficiency.
2. Pancreas—chronic pancreatitis—deficient secretion of pancreatic juice causes steatorrhoea with consequent weight loss (other cardinal signs are diabetes and calcification of the pancreas); really a failure of digestion rather than absorption in the small intestine.
3. Pancreas—fibrocystic disease of the pancreas (affects exocrine glands like the pancreas, bronchial, biliary and sweat glands with abnormally high Na content in sweat); causes steatorrhoea usually earlier in life than coeliac disease.
4. Protein-losing gastroenteropathy—abnormal loss of protein especially albumin through the stomach and intestine which may cause hypoalbuminaemia; seen with gastric carcinoma, regional enteritis, ulcerative colitis, congestive heart failure, etc.

Absorption

The surface area of the small intestine is increased by valvulae conniventes, also by numerous *villi* on the borders of which are *microvilli*. Absorption may be studied:

1. *in vivo*—disappearance of substances from lumen of gut of animals or man by balance experiments, e.g. radioactivity of urine and faeces following oral ^{58}Co vitamin B_{12} before and after the injection of intrinsic factor; oral fat intake compared with faecal fat excretion, etc.;
2. *in vitro*—especially using an isolated piece of rat intestine which has thrown light on some of the basic processes governing absorption, e.g. no absorption of water if glucose is absent; L-isomers of alanine, methionine, etc. are absorbed against a concentration gradient whereas the D-isomers are not (the main experimental technique now used employs an inverted sac of intestine).

These results indicate that absorption is an active process in the gastro-intestinal tract.

Sugars such as glucose and galactose are actively absorbed, but phosphorylation is no longer considered to be a prerequisite to absorption; dietary carbohydrates are mainly polysaccharides (starch, glycogen) or disaccharides (sucrose, lactose) and are hydrolysed by pancreatic amylase to mono- (mainly glucose) and disaccharides (mainly maltose, isomaltose). The disaccharides are split into monosaccharides in the plasma membrane of the microvilli (rather than by enzymes present in the succus entericus), and are then moved to the interior of the cells by an active transport system. Hence the secondary deficiency of disaccharidases in any condition which damages the mucosa (e.g. coeliac disease, tropical sprue), although a specific deficiency can occur, without obvious intestinal damage.

Fats are ingested as long-chain triglycerides and 90 per cent undergo hydrolysis in man before absorption (about 40 per cent completely hydrolysed to fatty acids and glycerol while the remainder are partially hydrolysed to mono- and diglycerides). These fats appear in the circulation after absorption as *chylomicrons* (formed in mucosal cells and they are a stable form of lipid; they are then transferred from the intestinal mucosal cells via the lymphatic system to the blood stream); medium- and short-chain fatty acids are absorbed into the portal system (but do not constitute an important factor in man).

Proteins can be absorbed intact in the newborn, but after this they are usually hydrolysed to peptides or amino-acids before absorption. Dietary proteins are split into amino-acids and simple peptides; the amino-acids are probably absorbed by utilising a specific carrier system in the intestinal mucosal wall. Defective amino-acid absorption can occur in cystinuria (L-lysine, ornithine, arginine are involved) possibly due to a disorder of a specific carrier in both renal tubular and jejunal epithelial cells. In Hartrup disease a similar situation exists for tryptophan and some related amino-acids.

Calcium.—There is a direct effect of vitamin D on active calcium transport.

Iron.—The mucosal block theory is now considered incorrect but the correct regulating mechanism governing iron absorption is not known.

Water.—Usually passively follows absorption of foodstuffs, and clinical difficulties with water absorption are usually due to altered particle absorption, e.g. diarrhoea in intestinal hyper-motility states where there is insufficient time for absorption of dissolved particles of hydrolysed food.

Vitamin B_{12}.—Binding of B_{12} by intrinsic factor secreted from the fundus and body of the stomach is an essential preliminary to its absorption from the distal part of the ileum (note that no other dietary component requires a specific alimentary tract secretion for its assimilation).

DISORDERS OF SMALL INTESTINAL ABSORPTION

In coeliac disease and its adult counterpart, idiopathic steatorrhoea, there is damage to the small intestine with disorganisation of the villi produced by the protein fraction, gluten, of various flours. This interferes with the absorption of many substances, e.g.:

food generally—growth ceases, wasting;

fats—diarrhoea, poor absorption of the fat-soluble vitamins, A, D;

glucose—flat oral glucose tolerance test (also abnormal absorption of D-xylose which is the basis of a clinical test for idiopathic steatorrhoea);

water—abnormal absorption can cause nocturnal diuresis;

vitamins—B-glossitis, stomatitis, cheilosis.

　　　　　　Folic acid and vitamin B_{12}—megaloblastic anaemia.

　　　　　　C—scurvy.

　　　　　　K—haemorrhage due to hypoprothrombinaemia.

　　　　　　D—rickets, tetany and osteomalacia.

A similar picture of a widespread disorder of absorption is seen in tropical sprue (unknown cause). All the above constitute *primary causes* of malabsorption, but there are *secondary causes* (commoner in the United Kingdom) due to:

1. gross organic disease of the digestive system, e.g. massive parasitic infestation (*Giardia lamblia*), regional enteritis, lack of bile (as in obstructive jaundice), lack of pancreatic enzymes (as in chronic pancreatitis);
2. reticulosis is an important cause;
3. gastro-intestinal surgery, e.g. after partial gastrectomy;

4. manifestation of a generalised disease, e.g. diabetes, systemic sclerosis;
5. chemicals and drugs, e.g. phenindione;
6. Zollinger-Ellison syndrome;
7. metabolic disorders, e.g. intestinal lactase deficiency, cystinuria.

Assessment of deficient small intestinal function in man

   (*a*) On clinical grounds—e.g.
       bulky pale stools of steatorrhoea;
       failure to regain normal weight after gastric surgery;
       osteoporosis, tetany;
       iron-deficiency anaemia refractory to iron therapy.

   (*b*) Laparotomy—allows recognition of focal disease, and is an early investigation particularly when pain is present.

   (*c*) Excess faecal fat—over 5 G. per day in stool on normal hospital diet.

   (*d*) X-ray, e.g.
       pancreatic calcification in chronic pancreatitis;
       gross intestinal disease such as diverticulosis of the small intestine, Crohn's disease, or clumping of barium in idiopathic steatorrhoea.

   (*e*) Faulty digestion or faulty absorption, e.g.
       glucose tolerance test—normal in pancreatic steatorrhoea, abnormal in idiopathic steatorrhoea;
       D-xylose excretion test—normal in pancreatic steatorrhoea, abnormal in idiopathic steatorrhoea;
       radioactive B_{12}—absorption—normal in pancreatic steatorrhoea, abnormal in idiopathic steatorrhoea and Addisonian anaemia.

   (*f*) Biopsy of the small intestine—abnormal mucosa in idiopathic steatorrhoea, coeliac disease, and helps make the correct diagnosis in Whipple's disease.

   (*g*) Dietary test—clinical response to gluten-free diet in children with coeliac disease (although this is no longer done by most clinicians).

COLON

Absorption.—Small amount of water daily; capacity to do this is relatively low (just over 2 litres per day in man) hence increased flow rate through the small intestine causes diarrhoea;

electrolytes—Na absorbed, also Cl (ureters transplanted into colon may cause hyperchloraemic acidosis);

bacteria break down protein products to indole, skatole, hydrogen sulphide (give faeces the characteristic odour) which are partly absorbed and detoxicated in the liver (see Chapter VIII);

divalent ions are not absorbed to any extent, e.g. magnesium sulphate holds water in the intestine and acts as a saline aperient.

Excretion.—Potassium is excreted so that diarrhoea can lead to hypokalaemia.

Defaecation

The desire occurs when faeces enters the rectum; afferent limb of the reflex arc (see Chapter X) is composed of parasympathetic nerves which go to the sacral part of the spinal cord, and the efferent fibres (parasympathetic) cause relaxation of the anal sphincters and contraction of the colonic muscle, (the emphasis is now on the relaxation of the sphincters rather than forceful peristalsis). There are also fibres to the cerebral cortex where control over the voluntary part of defaecation is exerted (this voluntary component of defaecation consists of the integrated relaxation of the external sphincter and contraction of the diaphragm and abdominal muscles ending with elevation of the pelvic floor and concomitant contraction of the sphincters which completes the expulsion). Normal defaecation is a complex act involving both voluntary and involuntary components. When the spinal reflex is abolished (e.g. injury to spinal cord, sacral nerves) defaecation is affected with initial severe constipation (and urinary retention) followed by "automatic" defaecation which occurs in the absence of any subjective sensations.

Abnormalities of colonic function.—Constipation and diarrhoea.

Constipation.—The term is used by patients in many different ways, but here refers to decreased frequency of defaecation. This may be acute (due to a severe febrile illness, an imperforate anus or acute intestinal obstruction), but the major causes are chronic as noted below:

1. voluntarily inhibiting the desire to defaecate because of convenience or a painful lesion around the anus;

2. physical inactivity, pregnancy;
3. weakness of the muscles involved in defaecation as in the debilitated and the elderly;
4. stasis in the colon due to slow movement of contents when there is a low level of roughage in the diet or in idiopathic megacolon;
5. obstruction:
    (a) outside the colon, e.g. pelvic tumour;
    (b) inside the colon, e.g. structural such as carcinoma; "physiological" such as absence of nerve plexuses or ganglia either congenital (Hirschsprung's) or acquired (Chaga's disease in which trypanosome parasites destroy the nerve ganglia in the walls of the colon);
6. chemicals and drugs, e.g. opiates, lead;
7. metabolic and endocrine causes, e.g. hypercalcaemia, porphyria, myxoedema;
8. abnormalities of the nervous system, e.g. higher voluntary control as in anorexia nervosa and depression, or lesions of the sacral roots.

Studies of colonic motility show that in some of the above conditions the colon is hyperactive, whereas in older patients with long history of constipation there may be reduced colonic motility.

Diarrhoea.—This may be due to causes arising in the small intestine as well as the colon:

Acute—infections, e.g. bacillary and amoebic dysentery (probably colon is also affected), cholera;
    ingested poisons or toxins;
    any cause of chronic diarrhoea may have an acute phase.
Chronic—gastro-intestinal causes—gastric causes, e.g. stomach operations;
    small intestinal causes, e.g. any cause of the malabsorption syndrome;
    colonic causes, e.g. carcinoma, ulcerative colitis, amoebic dysentery;
    non-gastro-intestinal causes—psychogenic, e.g. irritable colon syndrome; intraperitoneal infection, e.g. pelvic abscess; poisons and drugs, e.g. mercurials, broad-spectrum antibiotics; endocrine and metabolic, e.g.

thyrotoxicosis, diabetes, carcinoid syndrome, Zollinger-Ellison syndrome.

MOVEMENTS OF THE COLON

As in the small intestine, the main mechanism responsible for movement of colonic contents is relaxation of colonic muscle, and the so-called gastro-colic reflex is probably of no importance (if, indeed, it really exists). With rectal distension there is reflex inhibition of the tonically contracted external anal sphincter.

Irritable colon syndrome—a disorder of colonic behaviour in the absence of other evidence of organic disease, in which pain, diarrhoea or constipation may be present. The patient's personality and physical make-up seem to determine whether the colon bears the brunt of the reaction to stress (possibly with excess colonic activity with aggressive responses and vice versa with depressive responses). In many patients with the irritable colon syndrome there is increased colonic activity as shown by intraluminal pressure tracings; this overactivity represents resistance to transit of the contents and may contribute to the abdominal pain (detected by manometric studies). Colonic motility increases in both normal subjects and patients with the irritable colon syndrome with emotionally charged situations, but it is possible that the latter react excessively to para-sympathetic stimulation (increase in colonic activity after physostigmine greater than in normal person). Increased resistance to movement of colonic contents is seen in Hirschsprung's disease where there is a failure of relaxation of the abnormal bowel.

CLINICAL ASSESSMENT OF COLONIC FUNCTION

These methods are summarised below:

Inspection and rectal examination.
Sigmoidoscopy.
Barium enema.
Examine faeces.
Intestinal motility tests.

Chapter VIII

LIVER

BLOOD draining from the small intestine (portal venous blood) contains the products of digestion and it goes to the liver where synthesis of new products, alteration of toxic substances, storage and modification of food materials is undertaken.

Carbohydrate Metabolism

The liver converts dietary monosaccharides in the portal venous blood into glycogen which it stores (glycogenesis). Part of the total amino-acids metabolised in the body are converted into glycogen as well (gluconeogenesis), and the stored glycogen is converted into glucose (glycogenolysis) as required to keep the blood glucose level constant.

Normal formation and breakdown of glycogen:

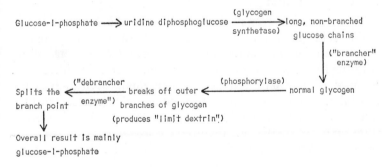

Glycogen storage disease.—A disorder of glycogen formation and deposition; there are several different forms:

(*a*) defective synthesis, e.g. deficiency of glycogen synthetase (which couples glucose molecules together to form glycogen); e.g. "brancher" enzyme deficiency (abnormal type of glycogen produced which is laid down in other organs as well as the liver);

(*b*) defective breakdown, e.g. glucose-6-phosphatase deficiency (von Gierke's disease): commonest type of glycogen storage disorder, unable to break down glycogen which is deposited in liver and kidneys, and there is hypoglycaemia; e.g. "debrancher" enzyme deficiency: like above but milder symptoms; e.g. myophosphorylase deficiency (McArdle's syndrome)—normal glycogen in muscles which cannot be properly metabolised but no hypoglycaemia; e.g. Pompe's disease—excess glycogen in the heart or muscles of no known cause.

Lipid Metabolism

The liver can synthesise fatty acids, and dietary fatty acids are transformed into the types more useful for metabolism. The liver also synthesises cholesterol and its esters from acetyl-CoA (see Chapter I) and produces cholic acid from the breakdown of cholesterol esters (the cholic acid is conjugated with glycine and taurine to make the bile salts): in addition the liver metabolises the steroids produced by various endocrine glands.

The metabolism of cholesterol is linked in some way to albumin synthesis for the hypoalbuminaemia of the nephrotic syndrome is accompanied by elevated blood cholesterol.

Protein Metabolism

The liver is involved in the formation of the "non-essential" amino-acids (i.e. those that can be made in the body and are not required in the food) and the final steps of nitrogen metabolism with the formation of urea and uric acid. In addition it forms a number of plasma proteins (e.g. albumin, fibrinogen, prothrombin and a major portion of the globulins). In foetal liver red cells are formed and this function can return after birth ("myeloid metaplasia") if the need for extramedullary (outside the bone marrow) sites of erythropoiesis arises.

Storage

The liver stores glycogen and also iron (as ferritin) and lipid-soluble vitamins (A, D) and vitamin B_{12}.

Detoxication

The liver is the site of most of those reactions which involve alteration of foreign materials which can be metabolised; this is done by acetylation (e.g. of aliphatic and aromatic amines), methylation, hippuric acid synthesis, oxidation and glucuronide and ethereal sulphate formation.

Excretory Role

Excretes bile which contains a variety of substances produced by or removed by the liver cells (including alkaline phosphatase excretion by an unknown mechanism).

BILE

A green alkaline fluid of mucoid consistency containing bile pigments, bile salts and cholesterol. It is produced continuously by the liver cells (500 – 700 ml. daily) and is stored and concentrated in the gall-bladder from which it is released intermittently to aid digestion of food. The passage of bile into the intestine is possible when the sphincter of Oddi (surrounds entrance of common bile duct into the duodenum) relaxes and the gall-bladder contracts under the influence of cholecystokinin (hormone released from upper small intestinal mucosa on contact with fat in intestinal lumen).

Bile salts are sterols, probably from cholesterol, and cholic acid is the most important constituent (conjugated with glycine or taurine): they help to emulsify fats and assist their hydrolysis (digestion). They also facilitate the action of pancreatic lipase and assist absorption of free fatty acids. Most of these bile salts are reabsorbed from the intestine, but the resin, cholestyramine, can pick up bile salts and remove them from the body (and consequently reduce the itching produced by bile salts in jaundice).

Bile pigments are derived from haemoglobin (see Chapter V) with bilirubin in the plasma being removed by the liver parenchymal cells, conjugated by glucuronyl transferase, and excreted in the bile as mono- and di-glucuronides. In the intestine bilirubin is broken down by bacteria to stercobilinogen which is mostly reabsorbed and re-excreted by the liver (*entero-hepatic* circulation), although a small amount is excreted in the urine as urobilinogen and a small amount is unabsorbed and excreted in the faeces to which it imparts the characteristic dark brown colour.

Some substances are actively secreted into bile:

e.g. bromsulphthalein (BSP)—used as test of liver excretory function; iodopanoic acid ("Telepaque")—used for X-ray visualisation of gall-bladder.

Liver Function Tests

These are based on the above metabolic functions of the liver which may become deranged in disease of the liver and biliary tree.

(a) Bilirubin metabolism—bilirubin glucuronides are water soluble, hence give the "direct" van den Bergh reaction with plasma (bilirubin itself is alcohol soluble giving the "indirect" reaction) (see below). Urinary urobilinogen is increased with increased hepatic excretion of bilirubin (haemolytic jaundice) and when the liver is damaged and unable to re-excrete urobilinogen absorbed from the intestine properly (an early sign in hepatocellular damage).

(b) Plasma proteins—in severe liver disease synthesis of albumin is impaired (may cause hypoalbuminaemia) while changes in the globulins in the serum account for the various flocculation and turbidity tests (zinc sulphate test depends on increased γ-globulin while thymol turbidity test depends on alteration in both β- and γ-globulins—see Chapter V on plasma proteins). There are often changes in γ-globulins in liver disease which can be detected by serum electrophoresis and these are an indication of the activity of cell damage.

(c) Clearance studies—depend on metabolism or excretion of some material which can be readily measured, e.g. bromsulphthalein (this dye is removed from the circulation by the liver cells and excreted into the bile).

(d) Enzyme studies—high blood levels of alkaline phosphatase occur in biliary obstruction; increased level of serum transaminase (especially SGPT) when the liver cells are damaged.

(e) Portal venous pressure—measured by a needle introduced into the spleen (normal 10 mm.Hg) and is a direct way of determining the presence of portal venous hypertension.

Jaundice.—Accumulation of bile pigments in body (detectable in sclera when plasma bilirubin over 2 mg./100 ml.); due to excess breakdown of haemoglobin (with consequent excess formation of bilirubin) or difficulty excreting bilirubin. In the liver parenchymal cell bilirubin in the plasma is transported to the ribosomes, conjugated with glucuronic acid (the enzyme involved is glucuronyl transferase), transported to bile canaliculi and excreted in the bile (note again that bilirubin glucuronides give direct van den Bergh reaction).

Classification:

(i) overproduction of bilirubin—excess unconjugated bilirubin in plasma (indirect van den Bergh reaction) due to increased red cell destruction (see Chapter V).

(ii) failure to transport bilirubin to the site of conjugation within liver cells—a congenital disorder sometimes called Gilbert's disease.

(iii) failure to conjugate bilirubin due to defective glucuronyl transferase activity (Crigler-Najjar syndrome and in neonatal jaundice when there is immaturity of the enzyme system).

(iv) failure to transport conjugated bilirubin to bile canaliculi —a brown pigment is deposited in the liver cells and there is a subnormal BSP clearance (Dubin-Johnson syndrome).

(v) intrahepatic obstruction to bile flow (cholestatic jaundice), e.g. some cases of virus hepatitis; due to drugs (commonest is chlorpromazine, then substituted testosterones).

(vi) extrahepatic obstruction to bile flow (obstructive jaundice) due to mechanical obstruction from stones in the common bile duct, carcinoma of the head of the pancreas.

CAUSES OF JAUNDICE

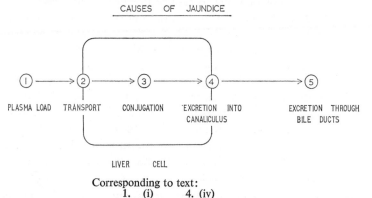

Corresponding to text:
1. (i)   4. (iv)
2. (ii)   5. (v) and (vi)
3. (iii)

(vii) diffuse damage to liver cells, e.g. due to acute virus hepatitis, cytomegalic inclusion disease, toxoplasmosis.

Blood supply.—Two separate systems give total blood supply of approx. 1·5l./min.

portal vein branches (80 per cent blood supply) ⎫
⎬ go to liver cells
hepatic artery branches (20 per cent blood supply) ⎭

while the central canals carry blood leaving the liver and join to form the hepatic venous system which empties into the inferior vena cava.

Portal venous system—a portal system has capillaries at both ends, and here capillaries in the gut drain to portal vein which divides into capillaries again in the liver. About 30 per cent of the portal venous blood comes from the spleen. The normal portal venous pressure averages 8 mm.Hg.

Portal hypertension.—Portal venous pressure may increase up to 50 mm.Hg in disease, and the increased pressure may lead to the formation of collateral vessels (e.g. oesophageal varices), which may rupture (causing gastro-intestinal haemorrhage), or distend the spleen (producing splenomegaly which may cause a leucopenia and thrombocytopenia—this condition is known as hypersplenism).

Causes—usually cirrhosis of the liver;
     thrombosis of portal or splenic veins.

It is sometimes possible to reduce portal venous pressure by anastomosing the portal vein to the inferior vena cava (porta-caval shunt) so that some blood bypasses the liver; however this may cause metabolic derangements leading to hepatic coma (a disturbance of consciousness seen in liver disease; in the earlier phases disorders of movement and changes in the E.E.G. occur). This coma is related to abnormal metabolism of nitrogenous products although it does not always correlate with an elevated level of blood ammonia (the liver normally forms urea from ammonia produced from amino-acid breakdown).

Ascites.—An ultra-filtrate of plasma which accumulates in the peritoneal cavity due to:

(*a*) portal hypertension—alone rarely causes ascites but needs hypoalbuminaemia also: however partly due to increase in capillary pressure with transudation of fluid according to Starling's Law of Capillaries (see Chapter IV);

(*b*) hepatic venous obstruction, e.g. thrombosis of hepatic veins; constrictive pericarditis;

(*c*) reduction in colloid osmotic pressure of plasma, e.g. reduced albumin synthesis when liver damaged by cirrhosis;

(*d*) increased secretion of aldosterone—removal of aldosterone from the blood by the liver is impaired in cirrhosis and there is a consequent increase in sodium retention by the kidney (see Chapter II) with increase in body water. This is never a primary cause of ascites but may be a contributing factor;

(*e*) increased permeability of the subperitoneal capillaries so that protein enters the peritoneal cavity from the plasma, e.g. malignant deposits on the peritoneum.

Chapter IX

THE KIDNEY

THE kidney has two main functions:
  (i) regulation of the body fluids;
  (ii) a humoral function (see Chapter II).

Anatomy

The functional unit is the nephron composed of a glomerulus and a tubule (a proximal convoluted section, then a long straight segment descending into and ascending out of the medulla called the loop of Henle, a distal convoluted tubule lying near the glomerulus and finally a collecting duct). The renal cortex is composed of glomeruli, proximal and distal convoluted tubules while the medulla contains the descending and ascending limbs of the tubules (loops of Henle) and the collecting duct system. The glomerulus is supplied by an afferent arteriole (which has the juxta-glomerular apparatus in its wall) and an efferent arteriole leaves the glomerulus and divides into the peritubular capillaries near the proximal tubule and these wind around the tubule along its length. Although the kidney receives a rich nerve supply, renal function does not appear to be modified by their action except under stressful situations, e.g. reduced renal blood flow on standing up; they do not appear to affect tubular function directly. As there is a large blood supply, the amount of oxygen extracted by the renal tissue is small per unit volume of blood (i.e. low arteriovenous oxygen difference). In an emergency, e.g. haemorrhage, the blood supply is drastically reduced.

Physiology

About one-fifth of the cardiac output goes to kidneys and the (almost) protein-free filtrate derived from the blood by the glomeruli is called the glomerular filtrate. It is identical with plasma except for this absence of protein and other colloids. In the tubule absorption and secretion of various substances occurs. The proximal tubule absorbs most of the filtered Na^+,

Cl', glucose, K$^+$ amino-acids and some HCO$_3'$, while the distal tubule and collecting ducts are engaged in the precise regulation of acid-base and K$^+$ balance. Some Na$^+$ is also reabsorbed in the distal tubule in exchange for H$^+$ and K$^+$ and ammonium ions.

Renal blood flow can be altered, e.g. following haemorrhage, by an active process, but in addition the isolated perfused kidney can keep flow fairly constant as the perfusing pressure is increased or decreased within certain limits. This is known as *autoregulation* and is thought to be due to a myogenic reflex. According to this theory the smooth muscle cells in the renal vasculature are said to respond to an increase in perfusion pressure by an increased strength of contraction.

The Concept of Clearance

The clearance value is an expression of the degree to which a substance is removed from the blood by excretion into the urine.

$$\text{Clearance} = \frac{\text{amount of substance in urine (per minute)}}{\text{concentration of substance in plasma}}$$

Inulin is freely filtered by the glomerulus and is not altered, reabsorbed or secreted by the nephrons. Its concentration in the plasma and glomerular filtrate are therefore identical. Hence in a steady state a knowledge of the amount leaving in the urine per unit time, and the plasma concentration at that time is sufficient to permit calculation of the rate of glomerular filtration (GFR). In clinical practice inulin is difficult to use and creatinine from normal metabolism is often used instead, i.e. endogenous creatinine clearance. A 24-hour urine specimen is collected and a plasma sample, and the creatinine content of each is determined. If the volume of urine is known the average creatinine clearance over a 24-hour period can be worked out. Urea clearance is sometimes used in man but, although it is related to glomerular filtration rate, it is not an accurate measurement of GFR because urea is partially reabsorbed by tubular cells. GFR in man is about 125 ml./min.

If a substance is *completely* removed from the plasma while passing through the kidneys then a knowledge of the clearance rate will be a measure of effective renal plasma flow. P-amino hippuric acid (PAH) is often used to measure this, and the plasma flow in man is about 650 ml./min.

The normal plasma urea and creatinine concentrations are 15 – 35 mg./100 ml. and about 1·0 mg./100 ml. respectively and as the clearance of these substances is dependent on the rate of glomerular filtration, it will be apparent that as filtration rate falls their plasma concentrations rise. Hence the use of blood urea and creatinine levels as a common test of renal damage in clinical medicine.

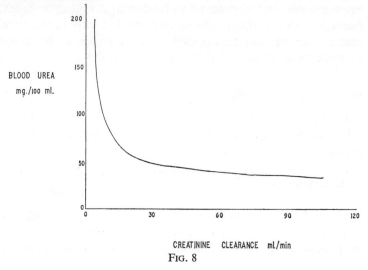

CREATININE   CLEARANCE   mL./min

Fig. 8

From the diagram it can be seen that as creatinine clearance falls, blood urea rises and there is rather a sharp curve in the graph. The clinical implication of this is that blood urea changes little until the filtration rate is very low, and then large changes in blood urea occur when an initial slight elevation of blood urea is subsequently followed by anything which produces a further small reduction in glomerular filtration rate, e.g. even a slight degree of heart failure. The blood urea is obviously not a sensitive indicator of moderate reduction in GFR due to renal damage. The following are causes of *impaired glomerular function*:

    (i) structural damage, e.g. acute nephritis, diabetic nephropathy;

   (ii) functional abnormality, e.g. shock, haemorrhage, Na^+ depletion, severe heart failure; obstruction to urine flow.

These may result in a retention of urea and other nitrogenous end-products of metabolism and a reduction in urine flow (ranging from oliguria to complete anuria). Glomerular damage may also cause a leak of plasma proteins and red cells into the urine, e.g. in glomerulonephritis.

Tubular Function

Some substances are absorbed while others are secreted into the urine by the renal tubular cells. These processes may be passive or active, usually the latter. Reabsorption of Na^+ and glucose, secretion of K^+ and PAH are active, while water and ammonia move passively. There is a maximum rate at which some substances can be moved across the tubular cells, known as the tubular maximum or Tm. This is the amount excreted in glomerular filtrate plus or minus amount present in the urine. When the process is operating at maximum capacity the maximum rate of transport for glucose averages 375 mg./min., and since the average GFR = 120 ml./min. it follows that the Tm will not be attained until the plasma concentration is about 300 mg. glucose/100 ml. In fact some glucose is found in the urine when the plasma concentration is over 200 mg./100 ml. due to all nephrons not being equal to their capacity to absorb glucose; i.e. "heterogeneity" of tubules. When glucose is found in the urine at lower plasma levels then there must be a disorder of tubular function, e.g. renal glycosuria, or the Fanconi syndrome when abnormal amino-aciduria is found as well as sugar in the urine. The common causes of glycosuria are associated with:

an elevated blood sugar—diabetes, thyrotoxicosis, Cushing's syndrome;
a normal blood sugar—renal glycosuria, Fanconi syndrome.

Tubular cells remove all the PAH presented to them by the blood up until a critical maximum value (Tm) and in man this is approx. 80 mg./min. and is a measure of the "tubular secretory capacity". This is not often used clinically.

The principal function of the proximal tubule is to reabsorb about two-thirds of the total solids and water from the glomerular filtrate (all the glucose, 90 per cent of Na^+ and Cl, most of the filtered K^+ and about half of the HCO_3'). Water moves freely with these substances so that the fluid in the proximal tubule remains isotonic to arterial blood. Na^+ is absorbed in exchange for H^+ as illustrated.

The rest of the filtrate is diluted by reabsorption of Na^+ and water in the ascending limb of Henle's loop. The distal convoluted tubule and collecting ducts may allow the hypotonic urine to pass out unchanged or else reconcentrate it. The

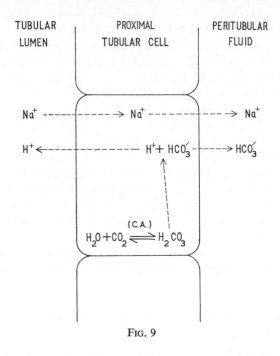

FIG. 9

ascending limb of the loop of Henle actively secretes Na^+ from the tubular fluid into the peritubular fluid, changing the osmolarity of the latter from the normal plasma level of approximately 280 milliosmols per litre in the cortex to a maximum of 1300 milliosmols/litre in the depths of the medulla (the counter current multiplier). Fluid inside the loop of Henle at the tip of the renal papilla is always *hypertonic* to normal plasma from mixed venous blood, and it is of the same solute concentration as the surrounding peritubular fluid while in the early part of the distal tubule it is hypotonic to plasma. These features are all due to active secretion of Na^+ by the ascending limb of the loop into the surrounding peritubular fluid. The ascending limb is also impermeable to water. Urea is probably treated similarly to Na^+, for urea is normally concentrated in the medulla as well as Na^+.

Fluid flowing down the collecting ducts will change its tonicity depending on the permeability of the cells of the collecting duct. Antidiuretic hormone (ADH—see Chapter II) renders the collecting duct permeable to water and water is absorbed into the hypertonic peritubular fluid and the urine is concentrated to a maximum of 1300 milliosmols/litre, equivalent to a urine specific gravity of 1·040. When ADH is absent dilute urine (hypotonic to plasma) is produced. Lack of ADH will cause diabetes insipidus (see Chapter II). Rarely the collecting duct cells fail to respond to the presence of circulating ADH, a condition known as vasopressin-resistant diabetes insipidus. The above mechanism for concentrating and diluting urine is known as the *counter current multiplier* (illustrated below).

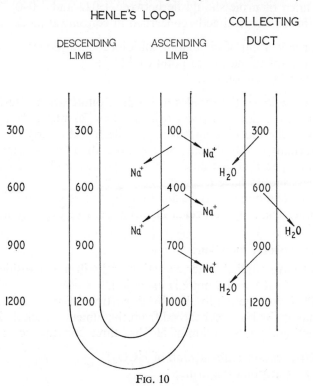

Fig. 10

Therefore circulating ADH and the functional integrity of the loop of Henle are essential for changing the osmolarity of the urine.

Clinically the concentration of the urine is measured by the specific gravity. This is actually related to the weight of solute in solution rather than the concentration of particles in solution, and may be erroneous in the presence of abnormally large molecules, e.g. sugar or the dyes used for intravenous pyelography (after intravenous pyelography urine specific gravity can rise to 1·060). The concentration is more correctly given by the osmolarity. The ability of the kidney to concentrate urine may be tested simply by determining the specific gravity of an early morning specimen of urine, or else a concentration-dilution study may be undertaken to determine the kidney's ability to handle water. The ability of the tubules to concentrate urine is tested by restricting all fluids for 24 hours (e.g. 8 a.m. one day to 8 a.m. the next morning when the specific gravity of at least one specimen of urine should lie between 1·022 and 1·040). There are three factors directly concerned in concentrating the urine:

concentration of circulating antidiuretic hormone;
ability of tubules to respond to ADH;
rate of solute output.

The capacity of the tubules to produce dilute urine is tested as follows: the fasting patient drinks water (20 ml./kg. body wt.) early in the morning and urine is collected at hourly intervals. A normal person should excrete more than three-quarters of the ingested fluid within the first four hours, and one specimen at least should have a specific gravity below 1·004. Inability to excrete a fluid load may be due to renal disease but could be due to other basically non-renal disturbances like hypoadrenalism.

Distal Tubular Functions

We have studied water excretion and will now consider H^+ ion, Na^+, K^+ and ammonia excretion.

H^+ is secreted into the distal portion of the nephron in exchange for Na^+ reabsorbed from the lumen, especially in the collecting duct. Secretion of H^+ has three consequences:

(i) it causes reabsorption of HCO_3';
(ii) it acidifies the urine;

(iii) is directly responsible for excretion of NH_4^+, by combining with NH_3 which has already diffused out of cells into lumen.

Sodium.—Most of the filtered Na_4^+ is reabsorbed in the proximal tubules by active transport as illustrated in Fig. 9. In the collecting ducts it is absorbed in exchange for K^+ and H^+ secreted by the tubular cells. Carbonic anhydrase is present in high concentration in the distal tubular cells and catalyses the formation of H^+ and HCO_3' from CO_2 and water, i.e. it helps provide a supply of H^+ ions for the $Na^+ - H^+$ exchange mechanism.

Ammonia is formed from glutamine and also from the deamination of amino-acids by the cells of the distal and

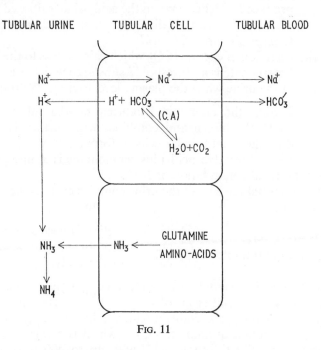

TUBULAR URINE   TUBULAR CELL   TUBULAR BLOOD

FIG. 11

collecting tubule. It can diffuse freely into the lumen where it accepts secreted hydrogen ions to become the ammonium ion. This cannot diffuse back and is therefore excreted in association with anions. In this way there is a further saving of metallic cations.

The Renal Regulation of Body pH

The processes by which the kidney is involved in controlling body pH are:

(i) conservation of HCO_3' by the kidney. Carbonic anhydrase helps produce H^+ and HCO_3' in tubular cells, and H^+ is excreted with subsequent absorption of Na^+. This leaves Na^+ and HCO_3' inside the luminal cells and they move into the blood from these cells. The collecting ducts are specialised for reabsorbing the remainder of the HCO_3' left in the tubular fluid, and Na^+ is absorbed here in exchange for H^+ and K^+, thus producing an acid urine. The H^+ secreted is coupled to Na_2HPO_4 to produce NaH_2PO_4. When the acid urine is titrated to the pH of blood with alkali, the amount of acid neutralised is called the *titratable acid*;

(ii) excretion of excess HCO_3' which gains access to the body. Bicarbonate is a "threshold" substance which is excreted in the urine when the plasma level exceeds 28 mEq/litre.

In addition the ammonia produced by the tubular cells diffuses into the lumen and combines with further H^+ ions excreted by the renal tubular cells to form ammonium ions. In fact, urinary titratable acid plus ammonium is a measure of the total renal conservation of Na^+.

On a normal mixed diet the urine contains every 24 hours the following:

25 mEq. NH_4
25 mEq. titratable acid
} Their excretion is necessary for the maintenance of normal acid-base balance of the body.

The kidney is the only way of excreting non-volatile acids formed by the metabolism of food. When excess acid is produced by the body, e.g. diabetic acidosis, there is a large increase in daily excretion of ammonium ion which is greater than the increase in daily titratable acid, with up to 400 mEq/24 hrs. urinary ammonium compared with 100 mEq/24 hrs. titratable acid. Both are increased in an attempt to conserve Na^+ (and hence HCO_3') for the body buffer stores. The lungs excrete as CO_2 the volatile acid H_2CO_3 formed by the metabolism of food.

The ability of the kidney to reduce the pH of urine can be

tested by giving oral ammonium chloride—i.e. by producing a metabolic acidosis. It is impaired in:

renal tubular acidosis (when the kidney is unable to produce a sufficient H^+ gradient between tubular cell and lumen); potassium deficiency (produces changes in histology of tubular cells); sometimes in hypercalcuria.

Renal Regulation of Body Na

The volume of the extracellular fluid is regulated by control of renal excretion of Na^+ and water (cf. osmolarity of ECF which is regulated by control of excretion of water by the posterior pituitary—see Chapter III). The mechanism for the regulation of ECF volume is not clear although the juxtaglomerular apparatus is one detector, and possibly also sensors in the right atrium are involved. The precise regulation of Na excretion depends on:

(i) haemodynamic alterations in the Na load presented to the renal tubules, e.g. 10 per cent fall in GFR in dogs can produce 50 per cent fall in Na excretion;

(ii) control of completeness of tubular reabsorption of Na by variations in the rate of excretion of aldosterone by the adrenal cortex (see Chapter II).

ACTION OF DIURETICS

A diuretic is a drug which produces an increased flow of urine, and the various types available will be discussed briefly here. To be useful clinically a diuretic must increase Na^+ output, i.e. cause a saluresis.

(i) Water produces a diuresis by inhibiting ADH secretion (see Chapter II) but is not used clinically for this purpose.

(ii) Osmotic diuretics, e.g. mannitol; the renal tubules are unable to reabsorb the diuretic from the glomerular filtrate in which it is dissolved and the material then exerts its own osmotic effect; there is an increased output of water and Na^+.

(iii) Acidifying salts, e.g. ammonium chloride; this is equivalent to administering HCl which is buffered by sodium bicarbonate and phosphate; if the Na^+ cannot be replaced rapidly enough by H^+ from the renal tubules, then excess Na^+ and water are excreted.

(iv) Xanthine diuretics, e.g. theophylline which increases GFR and reduces tubular reabsorption of Na^+ and water.

(v) Carbonic anhydrase inhibitors, e.g. acetazolamide ("Diamox") which decreases H^+ excretion by renal tubular cells, and hence there is less Na^+ reabsorption and increased Na^+ excretion in the urine. The Na^+ carries water with it.

(vi) The thiazide diuretics, e.g. chlorothiazide; inhibit Na^+ reabsorption by the renal tubular cells. They act directly upon renal tubular mechanisms involved in the transport of electrolytes between the tubular urine and the renal tubular cells. Part of their action is due to inhibition of carbonic anhydrase activity. They also increase K^+ secretion markedly.

(vii) Aldosterone antagonists, e.g. spironolactone; antagonise the action of aldosterone (see Chapter II) on the renal tubular cells and cause increased loss of Na^+ and Cl' with K^+ retention.

(viii) Mercurial diuretics, e.g. "Mersalyl"; inhibit Na^+ reabsorption especially by the proximal tubular cells.

(ix) Ethacrynic acid which blocks Na^+ and Cl' reabsorption in both proximal and distal renal tubules; also increases K^+ excretion (like the thiazides).

(x) Frusemide; main site of action on ascending limb of Henle's loop where Na^+ reabsorption is reduced.

Specific Tubular Defects

There are many specialised functions of the renal tubule which can go wrong either due to the influence of toxic substances or due to hereditary causes. Presumably the latter are often due to enzyme defects, usually with Mendelian recessive inheritance characteristics.

TOXIC (i) *exogenous poisons* may cause acute oliguric renal failure or, if less severe, may lead to multiple defects of tubular functions, e.g. heavy metal poisoning causes amino-aciduria, and glycosuria. A non-hereditary renal tubular acidosis (failure to excrete H^+ properly) can occur due to K^+-deficient nephropathy, chronic pyelonephritis and use of carbonic anhydrase inhibitors;

(ii) *endogenous poisons*—copper deposits in hepatolenticular degeneration cause amino-aciduria, glycosuria, hyperphosphaturia. Galactose-1-phosphate in galactosaemia causes amino-aciduria, occasional glycosuria and hyperphosphaturia.

HEREDITARY

Primary renal tubular acidosis is a congenital failure to excrete H^+ properly.

Congenital renal diabetes insipidus—collecting ducts unresponsive to circulating ADH (see Chapter II).

Renal glycosuria—tubular defect in which glucose appears in the urine in the presence of a normal blood sugar.

Cystinuria—disorder of tubular transport of the dibasic amino-acids cystine, lysine, arginine and ornithine which are excreted in the urine. There is a similar defect in the jejunal epithelium.

Hartnup disease—renal defect involving the excess excretion of amino-acids including alanine, serine, threonine, valine, leucine, phenylalanine, tyrosine, tryptophan and glutamine. There is also impaired intestinal absorption of tryptophan which accounts for the pellagra-like rash. Tryptophan is converted into nicotinic acid in the body and deficiency of nicotinic acid may cause pellagra (see Chapter XII).

Pseudohypoparathyroidism—the tubular cells are unresponsive to parathyroid hormone. Normally this hormone *inhibits* renal reabsorption of PO_4. Hence there is a high plasma $[PO_4]$ and low plasma [Ca] in this condition which is not influenced by injections of parathyroid hormone.

Idiopathic hypercalcuria—excessive calcium excretion with normal blood calcium level (a defect in renal Ca absorption).

Lignac-Fanconi syndrome—cystine deposited in various organs, including kidney, and renal tubular defects are of a generalised, non-specific character (glycosuria, amino-aciduria, reduced ability to excrete H^+ and NH_3).

Adult Fanconi syndrome—no cystine deposits but renal glycosuria, generalised amino-aciduria, reduced ability to excrete H^+ and excessive urinary K^+ loss. (Similar renal defects in Lowe's syndrome).

Hereditary vitamin D-resistant rickets—diminished ability of tubules to reabsorb phosphate, together with intestinal defects of Ca and PO_4 absorption.

RENAL FAILURE

Renal failure may be classified as either acute or chronic. Acute is usually taken as a sudden change in renal function which was previously normal, as compared to chronic renal failure which is a result of slowly progressive pathological changes in the kidneys. Uraemia ("urine in the blood") is a symptom complex resulting from the failure of renal function.

Acute renal failure.—Often defined by 24-hour urine volume excreted with sudden reduction to less than 720 ml. (some writers say down to less than 400 ml.), but more strictly it is acute renal insufficiency which does not permit the satisfactory excretion of urea and other products of protein metabolism which therefore accumulate in the blood. Hence acute renal failure can occur without oliguria. It may be caused by:

(i) Primary renal diseases—acute glomerulonephritis, acute pyelonephritis, obstructive renal disease, nephrotoxic agents.

(ii) Reduced blood flow—trauma, blood loss, serious systemic infections, water and salt depletion.

Although the major histological abnormality is usually in the renal tubular cells, glomerular filtration is also abnormal (i.e. tubular necrosis + reduced GFR leads to acute renal failure).

Physiological abnormalities important in therapy are:

inability to excrete water—hence restrict fluid intake to about 600 ml. plus any other loss, as for example vomit;

inability to excrete H^+ and metabolic acids—acidosis produced which reduces plasma $[HCO_3']$ and pH causes respiratory changes culminating in Kussmaul breathing (see Chapter IV);

inability to excrete nitrogenous products—increase in blood urea and creatinine;

inability to excrete K^+—this leads to an increase in plasma K^+ (can be detected by changes in the E.C.G. pattern for hyperkalaemia causes a high T wave and broad QRS especially) and this hyperkalaemia can lead to death. Reduction of plasma K^+ can be achieved by an insulin-glucose regime (which causes K^+ to pass from the blood back into body cells) and ion exchange resins; anabolic steroids may reduce the rate of rise of plasma K^+ from tissue catabolism (see Chapter II), but are not often used clinically.

If the above treatment will not prevent further deterioration then measures must be taken to remove metabolites from the body by peritoneal dialysis—using the peritoneum as a semi-permeable membrane or haemodialysis by machine.

The indications for dialysis are:

    clinical deterioration with mental confusion, muscle twitch-ing, acidotic breathing, blood urea over 300 mg./100 ml. or rapidly rising blood urea. Serum K^+ over 7 mEq/l. or HCO_3' below 12 mEq/l. (The actual levels of the above vary with the authority consulted.) In practice the indications vary more with the likely progression of the disorder related to the severity of trauma, etc. and with the pressure on the renal unit.

Chronic Renal Failure—due to:

  (i) destructive diseases of unknown cause, e.g. glomerulo-nephritis, polyarteritis nodosa, systemic lupus ery-thematosus;
  (ii) infection, e.g. pyelonephritis, tuberculosis;
 (iii) obstruction to urinary tract, e.g. bilateral ureteric calculi, prostatic hypertrophy;
 (iv) congenital lesions, e.g. polycystic kidneys;
  (v) hypertension;
 (vi) others, e.g. gout, amyloid, diabetic nephropathy, myelomatosis, radiation nephritis.

In all forms of chronic renal disease there is a diminished number of functioning nephrons, so that the solute load per nephron is increased. Hence, if urea production is constant, as nephrons are destroyed and GFR falls, the excretion of urea will fall and the blood urea will rise until a new steady state is achieved. The blood urea will increase if there is any further

fall in GFR (see Fig. 8), or there is increased urea production
due to an increase in food intake or tissue catabolism, e.g. due
to infection.

The earliest change in chronic renal failure is impairment of
the ability to concentrate urine, probably due to increased load
of solute per nephron, but in pyelonephritis there is also destruction of those parts of the nephrons responsible for
concentrating the papillary interstitial fluid and this may also
contribute. Later there is difficulty excreting a water load
because there are too few nephrons (watch for water intoxication
in advanced renal failure when given excess water to reduce
azotaemia) (*azotaemia* is the presence of increased concentrations of nitrogenous waste products in the blood).

Sodium and potassium.—Ability to excrete excess Na$^+$ is
limited: occasionally the kidney is unable to conserve Na on a
restricted intake (if Na$^+$ loss becomes severe this can reduce the
GFR and produce a further increase in azotaemia). K$^+$
excretion is well maintained until the terminal stage of renal
failure.

Acidosis.—Fall in plasma [HCO$_3'$] due to inability to excrete
acid which has to be buffered to prevent change in blood pH.
Rarely associated with an increased plasma [Cl$'$]. Reduction in
ammonia and titratable acid excreted causes the uraemic
acidosis.

Calcium and phosphorus.—Diminished excretion of phosphate
causes an increased plasma phosphate and there may be reduction in plasma Ca$^+$. Resistance also develops to the effect of
vitamin D on the intestine (i.e. one possible cause of a reduced
Ca absorption).

Chronic renal failure has the following phases:

(i) diminished renal reserve—about half of the nephrons
have been destroyed; there is no detectable abnormality
on ordinary examination or positive investigations;

(ii) renal insufficiency—mild azotaemia on normal diet;
impairment in urine concentration; certain stresses may
precipitate more marked renal failure, e.g. cardiac
failure associated with the hypertension often found;
infections, obstruction by calculi;

(iii) renal failure—more severe azotaemia with acidosis,
hyponatraemia, hyperphosphataemia, but without any
particular symptoms;

(iv) uraemia—symptoms and signs due to deranged renal function. These are not due to excess urea but to unknown toxins in the blood. The clinical features of uraemia include anorexia, mental disturbances, muscle twitching and pericarditis.

Chronic renal failure may be treated by:

remedying any factors producing sudden decompensation, e.g. by surgery or correcting salt depletion, shock or renal infection;

reducing azotaemia by restricting dietary protein intake (e.g. down to 40 G. protein daily);

alkali for severe acidosis, e.g. oral sodium bicarbonate;

treating the terminal hyperkalaemia (as for acute renal failure);

renal osteodystrophy is commonly symptomatic in adults (bone pain may be a troublesome symptom) and is treated by giving sodium bicarbonate if the blood pressure is not raised;

correcting the anaemia (which is due to defective erythro-poiesis and increased haemolysis) by blood transfusion (it is necessary to give packed red cells slowly to avoid raising the blood urea or precipitating cardiac failure);

chronic dialysis and/or renal transplantation.

Investigations in renal disease—in summary:

(a) Blood levels of metabolites, e.g. urea, creatinine.

(b) Plasma electrolyte concentrations.

(c) Clearance studies, e.g. endogenous creatinine clearance.

(d) Measuring the concentrating power, e.g. specific gravity of early morning specimen.

(e) Specific tests of tubular function, e.g. acid loading test for estimating H^+ excretion, chromatography for amino-aciduria.

(f) Differential renal function tests for unilateral renal disease, e.g. measure creatinine, Na^+, PAH excretion and specific gravity of urine from each kidney separately.

Chapter X

THE NERVOUS SYSTEM

THE PROPERTIES OF EXCITABLE MEMBRANES

THERE is an unequal distribution of ions across the cell membrane in any animal tissue, and in man there is a high concentration of K^+ inside the cell (low outside) and a high concentration of Na^+ outside in the interstitial fluid (low inside the cell). There is an electrical potential across the cell membrane (detectable when a fine electrode is pushed across the cell membrane) as high as 90 millivolts (mV) (inside negative to outside) in skeletal muscle cells and nerve cells—the *resting potential*.

CELL MEMBRANE

The cell membrane plays an important part in maintaining these ionic differences. Although Na^+ and K^+ ions can move across the cell membrane, any Na^+ which enters the cell is actively pumped out (i.e. this is a process that requires energy), and it is this *active transport* of Na^+ which keeps intracellular $[Na^+]$ low and intracellular $[K^+]$ high (Na^+ pumping is probably coupled to equal uptake of K^+; Na^+ and K^+ appear to be passed through the cell membrane by "carriers" limited to the membrane but the nature of the carrier system is unknown).

It is because of the unequal distribution of ions that the nerve cell develops and maintains a steady transmembrane electrical potential. The membranes of nerve and muscle cells possess the distinctive property of being *excitable*. An environmental change, or stimulus, produces a *transient depolarisation*, usually by increasing the permeability of the membrane to Na^+ or to Na^+ and K^+. Depolarisation is followed rapidly by a spontaneous recovery or repolarisation process which restores the original ionic state. This sequence of changes produces the nerve impulse and the accompanying voltage change is called an *action potential.* In the long thin nerve cell the impulse travels from the stimulus site to adjacent regions of the membrane—known as *self-propagation*—and hence can convey information from one part of the body to another.

Stimulus.—There is a minimal strength of stimulus, the threshold, necessary to evoke a propagating action potential, and one less than this, a sub-threshold stimulus, has only a local

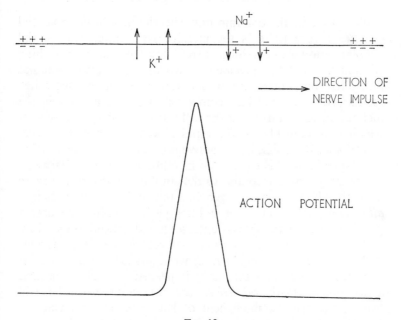

FIG. 12

(non-propagated) effect. A local, non-propagated or electrotonic potential causes:

transient increase in Na^+ permeability;
increased K^+ efflux;

and the potential charge later returns to normal.

An above-threshold stimulus produces a vast increase in Na^+ permeability and large influx of Na^+ with local depolarisation of the nerve cell membrane and an action potential (the Hodgkin cycle); there is a change in intracellular potential (with reference to extracellular fluid) from, say, -90 mV. to $+40$ mV., i.e. an action potential of 130 mV. is produced.

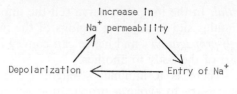

THE HODGKIN CYCLE

Note that in the diagram opposite the membrane potential changes before there is the massive Na^+ influx (this initial depolarisation is due to local current flow from the approaching stimulus). The Na^+ movement across the nerve membrane has fallen to about one-sixth of its peak value at a time when repolarisation is only half completed. There is a delay in the increase in K^+ efflux from the cell but it is this K^+ movement which is responsible for the rapid repolarisation of the nerve membrane. K^+ efflux is still above normal when repolarisation is complete and this causes the membrane to hyperpolarise.

The propagated response to the stimulus is always the same no matter how much stronger than threshold the stimulus is— *all-or-none* behaviour. For a brief period during the action potential it is impossible to elicit a second action potential no matter how strong the stimulus (when Na^+ influx is still present) —the *absolute refractory period*, while just after this period a stimulus greater than threshold is needed to excite a second action potential—the *relative refractory period* (when K^+ is still leaving the cell the movement of Na^+ needed for an action potential will be greater than normal). The length of the refractory period will determine the rate of impulse discharge in nerve fibres (as indeed it does in the heart where it limits the rate at which ventricular muscle will respond to a very rapid stimulus).

Electric currents flow between the active area of nerve and inactive region ahead of the nerve impulse—*local circuit currents*, and these increase the permeability of the adjacent nerve membrane to Na^+ and permit propagation of the nerve impulse along the nerve fibre (which is really part of a grossly elongated cell).

In myelinated nerves there is a much greater speed of impulse conduction for the impulse skips from one unmyelinated area (node of Ranvier) to the next (*saltatory conduction*), i.e. the myelin sheath (which is formed by Schwann cells) acts as an insulator with occasional breaks at the nodes of Ranvier. Resting and action potentials are only generated at these nodes in myelinated nerves.

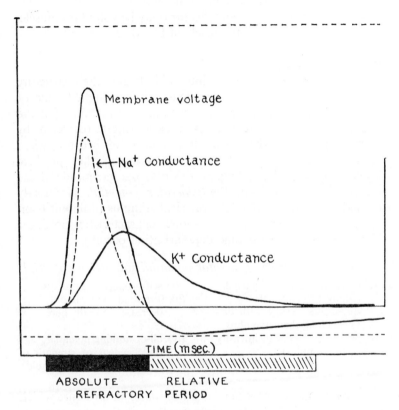

FIG. 13

The largest nerve fibres conduct at the greatest velocity and there is a relationship between intranodal length (between nodes of Ranvier), fibre diameter and conduction velocity in a nerve fibre. Saltatory conduction of a nerve impulse is probably rapid because the time taken for membrane depolarisation is reduced as most of the nerve is covered with a rapidly conducting myelin sheath.

THE REFLEX ARC

The basic unit of organisation in the central nervous system is the *reflex arc* which consists of two parts:

(i) sensory receptor and afferent nerve fibre;

(ii) efferent nerve fibre to effector (may be voluntary muscle, or gland or smooth muscle of blood vessel, etc.).

Sensory Receptors

These may respond to various stimuli and their structure varies accordingly. Stimuli detected vary from light (retina of eye), heat, chemicals, etc. to mechanical distortion of nerve endings and finally changes in muscle length (detected by muscle spindles). These stimuli are effective because when applied to appropriate afferent fibre terminals they produce *depolarisation* of the ending. In this case the magnitude of the resultant depolarisation, the *generator potential*, is directly related to the intensity of the physical stimulus (different from nerve fibres where an all-or-none characteristic produces identical response each time depolarisation occurs).

Differences between *generator potential* and *action potential:*

(i) stationary, non-propagated	(i) self-propagating process
(ii) confined to terminals	(ii), (iii) conducted without decrease along the fibre
(iii) diminishes rapidly with distance along the nerve fibre	
(iv) graded (varies with intensity of the stimulus)	(iv) all-or-nothing potential (independent of strength of stimulus if above threshold)

i.e. the sensory receptor acts as a *transducer* (a structure which converts one kind of energy into another, in this case converts pressure, light, chemical stimuli, etc. into electrical energy). The frequency of the spike discharge in the nerve fibre from a sensory receptor is related to the generator potential which, in turn, is related to the strength of the applied stimulus.

Increase in the strength of stimulus applied to a sensory receptor causes an increase in the frequency of action potentials propagated along the nerve fibre from the receptor. In this way the body is better able to determine the state of the external environment and also the internal state of the body. This applies to the determination of muscle length (by muscle spindles), position of joints (variety of receptors) and also the arterial blood pressure (carotid sinus and aortic arch presso-receptors) or the distension of the lungs (stretch receptors and the basis for the Hering-Breuer reflex—see Chapter VI).

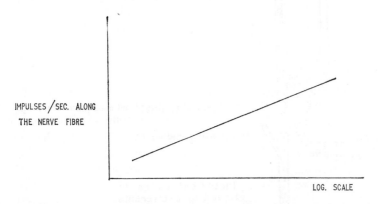

IMPULSES / SEC. ALONG THE NERVE FIBRE

LOG. SCALE

INTENSITY OF STIMULUS APPLIED TO SENSORY RECEPTOR

Stretch Receptor

In view of its importance in understanding muscle tone and posture, and as a basis for a number of clinical tests, the stretch receptor and stretch reflex will be described in detail.

The muscle spindle consists of endings to detect muscle length (annulospiral endings, flower-spray endings), together with special (intrafusal) muscle fibres (which are specially innervated by γ-efferent nerve fibres from the spinal cord) which can be caused to contract independently of the ordinary, or extrafusal, muscle fibres (the intrafusal fibres lie parallel to the origin and insertion of the extrafusal fibres); hence the intra-fusal fibres can change the tension on the annulospiral and flower-spray endings independent of any changes in the length of the muscle. Therefore, muscle spindles can detect change in length of a particular muscle in the body, and the threshold (or sensitivity) of this detecting system can be changed by the γ-efferent nerves to the muscle spindle.

The discharge along the γ-efferent nerves which go from the spinal cord to the muscle spindle (and change the sensitivity of the muscle spindle) is regulated by descending tracts in the spinal cord coming from various areas in the brain.

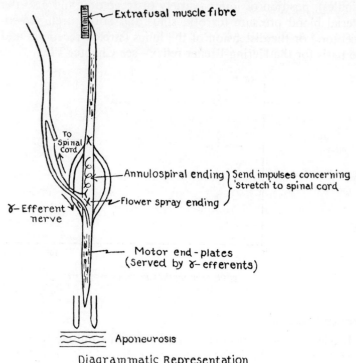

Diagrammatic Representation
of Muscle Spindle

FIG. 14

The muscle spindles can detect changes in the length of the muscle and their threshold can be changed by stimulation by the γ-efferent nerve fibres from the spinal cord; this is illustrated below:

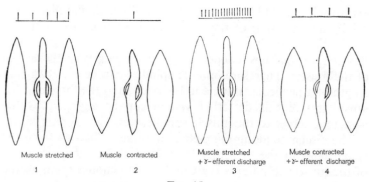

FIG. 15

The Stretch Reflex

Considering the simplest reflex in the body, namely the *stretch* reflex, there are the following components:

- (*a*) receptor (the endings of the muscle spindle $\big\langle$ annulospiral flower-spray) and the afferent nerve to the spinal cord;
- (*b*) the motor neurone in the spinal cord which conducts impulses to the effector organ (in this case voluntary muscle).

There is only one break (synapse) in the continuity of the nerve pathway—in fact the stretch reflex is a *monosynaptic* reflex. A good example of the stretch reflex is the knee jerk—tapping the patellar tendon in man causes contraction of the extensors of the knee (which then "jerks"). Tapping the patellar tendon stretches the muscle spindles in the knee extensor muscles and this information is carried back to the spinal motor-neurones supplying the extensor muscles of the knee, which then contract. The main reflexes of this type studied in man are:

the jaw jerk;
the biceps jerk;
the triceps jerk;
the supinator jerk;
the knee jerk;
the ankle jerk.

Reduction or absence of these reflexes means some disorder of the nerves, the effector organ (the muscle), or changes in impulses from higher centres in the central nervous system which play on the reflex arc.

Disorders of the Reflex Arc

- (i) Disease affecting the afferent pathway, e.g. tabes dorsalis (affects the posterior spinal nerve roots);
- (ii) diseases affecting the efferent pathway, e.g. poliomyelitis or motor neurone disease which damage the cell body of the efferent nerve fibre; polyneuritis (degeneration of the motor nerve fibre to muscle);
- (iii) diseases affecting the effector organ, namely the muscle, e.g. the myopathies;

(iv) diseases affecting impulses from higher centres (i.e. upper motor neurone lesions which are dealt with later).

COMMONEST CLINICAL CAUSES OF DIMINISHED TENDON REFLEXES

tabes dorsalis	diabetes mellitus
polyneuritis	poliomyelitis
Holmes-Adie syndrome	damage to nerve fibres by vertebral
syringomyelia	disc disease, e.g. sciatica, cervical
	spondylosis
congenital absence	old age

In addition the tendon reflexes enter the spinal cord at different levels and specific alteration of these reflexes can help in the determination of the anatomical position of certain disorders, e.g. a tumour compressing nerve roots in the region of the spinal cord.

The basic anatomical arrangement of the reflex arc is as illustrated in Fig. 16.

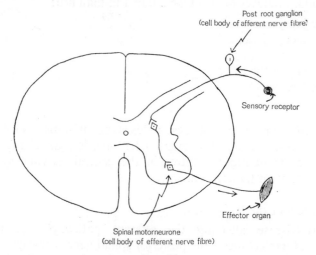

Post root ganglion (cell body of afferent nerve fibre?)

Sensory receptor

Effector organ

Spinal motorneurone (cell body of efferent nerve fibre)

FIG. 16

The *flexor* reflex—when a noxious stimulus (e.g. a pin prick) is applied to the foot of a spinal animal the leg is flexed (spinal animal is used to remove impulses from higher centres which may complicate the study of these reflexes). Sherrington called this reflex a nociceptive reflex because the stimulus applied is harmful to the tissues: such a flexor reflex has been described in man by Babinski—when spinal motor neurones to the leg are deprived of their cerebral control by the pyramidal tract, a noxious stimulus applied to the foot (e.g. a key stroked across the sole of the foot) causes the big toe to extend and the toes fan out, and when fully developed there is flexion of all joints in the lower limb (Oppenheimer's reflex occurs when a noxious stimulus, namely moving pressure over the tibia, is applied causing the same flexor response; it is physiologically similar to the Babinski reflex). The presence of the Babinski or Oppenheimer reflex in man indicates a lesion of the cortiocospinal (pyramidal) tract, e.g.

(i) precentral cerebral tumour;
(ii) damage to the pyramidal tract in internal capsule or brain stem (as occurs in cerebrovascular disease, i.e. a "stroke");
(iii) spinal cord compression, e.g. cervical spondylosis, spinal cord tumour;
(iv) spinal cord degeneration, e.g. disseminated sclerosis, subacute combined degeneration of the spinal cord (vitamin B_{12} deficiency—see Chapter V), hereditary ataxia (e.g. Friedreich's ataxia);
(v) it may also be present bilaterally in coma, normal sleep and hypoglycaemia.

If the stimulus is increased then reflex withdrawal of the stimulated limb is associated with contraction of the extensor muscles of the opposite limb—the *crossed extensor reflex*. If the stimulus leads to greater irradiation in the spinal cord (e.g. some months after spinal transection in man) one may even see a *mass reflex* response associated with withdrawal of both extremities, sweating, defaecation and urination following a vigorous scratch to the plantar surface of the foot.

Other clinically important reflexes are:

the grasp reflex—present in babies, but its occurence on one side in an adult later in life suggests a lesion of the opposite frontal lobe;
superficial abdominal reflexes—reduction means damage to the corticospinal tract;

jaw jerk—example of stretch reflex (stretching of muscle supplying mandible);

corneal reflex—noxious stimulus to cornea detected by cranial nerve V causes contraction of orbicularis oculi;

light reflex—light into eye detected by retina; visual pathways connect with III cranial nerve nucleus and lead to pupillary contraction: its absence in neurosyphilis is probably due to a lesion in the ciliary ganglion and is the basis of the Argyll Robertson pupil (which reacts normally on accommodation as fibres by-pass ciliary ganglion and so escape damage);

autonomic reflexes—seen in the mass reflex in spinal man.

SPINAL CORD ORGANISATION

Composed of:

central grey matter—nerve cell bodies and nerve fibres (mostly non-myelinated);

peripheral white matter—only nerve fibres (myelinated and non-myelinated).

There are areas of the spinal cord which subserve specific functions:

(*a*) ascending (sensory) tracts;

(*b*) descending (motor) tracts.

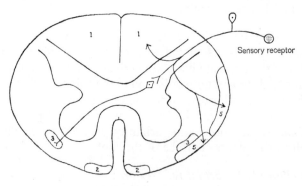

Sensory receptor

Fig. 17

Ascending Tracts

1. Ascending tracts of gracilis and cuneatus—convey sensation of:

posture;
passive movement;
vibration sense;
some light touch;

from sensory receptors in the upper and lower limbs. Terminate in nuclei (gracilis and cuneatus) in medulla: synapse there and 2nd fibres cross to the opposite side (sensory decussation), and ascend as the medial lemniscus to end in thalamus.

2. Ventral spinothalamic tract—sensory fibres synapse in posterior horn of grey matter and 2nd fibre crosses to opposite ventral spinothalamic tract: end in thalamus. Convey touch sensations.
3. Dorsal spinothalamic tract (similar path to 2): conveys pain, heat, cold sensations.
4. Pain, heat and cold sensation from face goes via 5th cranial nerve (trigeminal) to ipsilateral nucleus in medulla, and 2nd fibre crosses over and ends in thalamus.
5. Spinocerebellar tracts (dorsal and ventral)—convey proprioceptive impulses to the cerebellum.

From the optic thalamus fibres run to postcentral gyrus of cerebral cortex (partly to precentral gyrus), but the sensory functions of the cortex only involve the following sensations (on the opposite side of body):

appreciation of positional and passive movement at joints;
recognition and accurate localisation of light touch;
tactile discrimination and appreciation of size, shape, texture;
discrimination of different degrees of heat and cold.

The optic thalamus appears to be the end-station for the appreciation of the qualitative aspects of pain, heat, cold.

The modes of sensation investigated clinically are: light touch and tactile localisation, pressure touch, superficial and deep pain, temperature, sense of position and detection of passive movement at joints, vibration, discrimination between stimulation of two areas of skin simultaneously and appreciation of shape and form.

CLINICAL DISTURBANCES OF SENSATIONS

Lesions involve:

(a) *Peripheral nerves.*—Sensory symptoms in distribution of affected nerve:

incomplete lesions lead to paraesthesiae (e.g. numbness, tingling), e.g. cervical spondylosis (usually altered light touch and tactile discrimination in upper limb due to osteophytes projecting into the intervertebral foramina and pressing on nerve roots);

carpal tunnel syndrome where there is compression of the median nerve;

lateral cutaneous nerve of thigh constricted by fibrous tissue causing meralgia paraesthetica;

complete lesions, e.g. fractured humerus damaging the radial nerve;

meningovascular syphilis and tabes dorsalis;

extramedullary tumours;

herpes zoster (acute virus infection which attacks dorsal root ganglia);

vertebral collapse (primary or secondary neoplasm, tuberculosis or other infection, Paget's osteitis or traumatic fracture or dislocation);

intervertebral disc lesions (especially cervical and lumbar regions of spine, the latter often causing sciatica).

POLYNEURITIS—impaired function of many peripheral nerves due to following:

Guillain-Barré syndrome;

acute infectious polyneuritis;

alcholism;

diabetes;

lead poisoning;

vitamin B_1 or B_{12} deficiency;

diphtheria;

and a number of rarer causes (ranging from collagen diseases to leprosy).

(b) *The spinal cord.*

Brown-Séquard syndrome—A lesion limited to one half of the spinal cord causes: loss of appreciation of posture, passive joint movement, vibration sense and tactile discrimination on *same* side below lesion (destruction post-columns); analgesia and thermo-anaesthesia on *opposite* side of body (due to destruction of lateral spinothalamic tract);

(because there is a double route of fibres for light-touch and tactile localisation there is no loss of these sensations from unilateral cord lesion).

Tabes dorsalis—degeneration of post-columns with loss of appreciation of posture, passive movement, tactile discrimination and vibration.

Subacute combined degeneration—as for tabes and due to vitamin B_{12} deficiency (see Chapter V).

Syringomyelia—central cavitation of the cord causing "dissociated sensory loss" (loss of pain, heat and cold but not other sensations—note relation of fibres crossing to opposite spinothalamic tract below central canal of cord).

(*c*) *The brain stem.*—The commonest specific lesion here is thrombosis of the posterior inferior cerebellar artery causing:

hemi-analgesia and thermal anaesthesia *opposite* side of body, hemi-analgesia and thermal anaesthesia *same* side of face (also vertigo and cerebellar deficiency, involvement of nucleus ambiguus, and Horner's syndrome as these areas are supplied by same artery).

(*d*) *Optic thalamus.*—Gross impairment of all forms of sensibility on the opposite side of the body. May be "thalamic over-reaction" after vascular lesions with sensation of discomfort, heat and cold on opposite side of body.

(*e*) *Sensory cortex.*—Destructive lesions causing loss of appreciation and localisation of light touch; loss of two point discrimination, inability to determine shape, size or form in three dimensions (astereognosis); also may be sensory inattention or extinction;

irritative lesion, e.g. epileptic discharging lesion producing numbness or tingling opposite side of body.

DESCENDING TRACTS

1. Dorsal (indirect) corticospinal (pyramidal) tract from cerebral cortex: crosses to opposite side in medulla: goes to anterior horn cells (motor neurones). The fibres of the tracts are derived from cells in areas of the cortex which includes the precentral gyrus and are not only the axons of pyramidal cells. There are many more fibres in the pyramidal tract than there are Betz cells in the precentral gyrus.

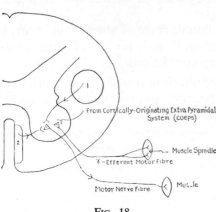

FIG. 18

2. Ventral (direct corticospinal tract: as for 1 except represents about 10 per cent of the pyramidal tract fibres which do not cross in the medulla).
3. There are many other descending tracts which connect with anterior horn cells and influence muscle contraction, but their specific functions are not yet clearly delineated—they include:

vestibulospinal—impulses conveyed from vestibular nuclei;
tectospinal—both the retina and the ear send fibres to the superior and inferior colliculus and from here impulses descend to influence the spinal motor neurones;
reticulospinal—comes from cells scattered through the reticular formation of the brain stem and goes to spinal motor neurones (both those to voluntary muscle and also to the cells of γ-efferents which are involved in altering muscle spindle tone and hence the threshold for response—see earlier section).

CLINICAL DISTURBANCES OF DESCENDING PATHWAYS

A lesion directly involving the efferent path of the reflex arc is often called a lower motor neurone disorder while that affecting pyramidal and extrapyramidal tracts going to the spinal motor neurone is called an upper motor neurone disorder. These can be differentiated clinically:

UMN lesion	*LMN lesion*
No wasting	Wasting of muscles
Increase in muscle tone	Flaccidity of muscles
Increased tendon reflexes	Reduced or absent tendon reflexes

Upper motor neurone lesions may originate in:

(a) Cerebral cortex—often only monoplegia and can cause Jacksonian epilepsy, e.g. cerebral tumour.

(b) Subcortical—in corona radiata upper motor neurones converge towards the internal capsule so that lesions here involve more fibres than cortical lesions of same size (hence causes a more severe clinical disability than would a similar sized lesion affecting the cerebral cortex).

(c) Internal capsule—fibres crowded together and lesion likely to produce a severe contralateral hemiplegia, e.g. haemorrhage.

(d) Brain stem—as both corticospinal tracts close may produce quadriplegia; other brain stem lesions include a unilateral cranial nerve plasy with a contralateral hemiplegia.

(e) Spinal cord—no involvement of cranial nerves: if the lesion is above cervical enlargement both legs and arms involved, but if below, then only legs affected.

Muscle Tone

In clinical practice muscle tone is tested by the resistance of muscle to passive elongation or stretch. Sherrington considered that it is concerned in maintaining posture, but electromyographic findings in healthy man reveal no electrical events occurring in most muscles which are involved in maintaining posture when the individual is in a standing position. In spite of this, conventional physiological teaching is that the fundamental basis of tone is the myotatic or stretch reflex mentioned previously. It is probable that the visco-elastic properties of muscle are of importance in determining muscle tone. The physiological (as opposed to clinical) idea is that on the background of tone established through the stretch reflexes, there are influences from higher centres which affect the spinal motor neurones involved (and also the γ-neurones which regulate the sensitivity of the muscle spindle): hence the spinal motor neurone has been referred to as the *"final common path."*

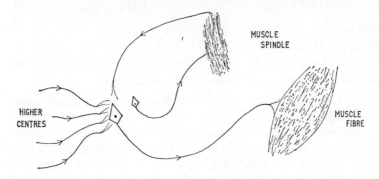

The higher centres involved in affecting the spinal motor neurones involved in the stretch reflex (and hence muscle tone) are:

labyrinth and muscle receptors in the neck;
cerebellum;
midbrain;
cerebral cortex.

When a lesion occurs in the midbrain in man a state of *decerebrate* rigidity may be produced (sustained contraction of the extensor muscles with rigid extension of all four limbs) and this is due to removal of inhibitory influences on the stretch reflex from higher centres.

Factors affecting muscle tone:

cerebellum—cerebellar deficiency can produce hypotonia;
reticular formation—removal of its influence causes decerebrate rigidity;
corticospinal tract—damage to it causes increased tone. This is the "classical" story but experimental damage to area 4 of the cerebral cortex in animals (in front of the fissure of Rolando and containing the giant pyramidal or Betz cells) and the pyramidal tract causes flaccidity rather than spasticity and spasticity is due to interruption of COEP fibres. (The "cortically originating extrapyramidal system" or COEPS is composed of extrapyramidal pathways from cerebral cortex to spinal cord which differ from the pyra-

midal or corticospinal system: COEPS is not a synonym for
"extrapyramidal system" but refers to that portion of it
which originates in the cerebral cortex);

lower motor neurone, i.e. reflex arc damage causes hypotonia
by interfering with the reflex arc;

similar effect from lesions affecting the muscles themselves.

These influences can be summarised as follows:

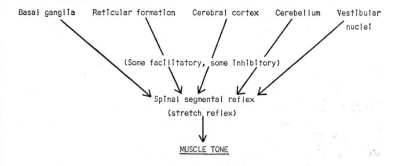

CLINICAL DISORDERS OF MUSCLE TONE

Hypotonia—(i) seen in cerebellar disorders, after an acute
lesion of one cerebral hemisphere or the spinal
cord ("neural shock");

(ii) chorea—a disorder of the basal ganglia;

(iii) lesion on afferent side of reflex arc, e.g. tabes
dorsalis;

(iv) lower motor neurone lesions (interrupt spinal
reflex arc like (iii) except that the efferent side
is involved);

(v) primary muscle degeneration, e.g. the myopathies.

Hypertonia—regarded as a "release" phenomenon (i.e. it is
due to the removal of some controlling influence on tone).

A clinical lesion which interrupts the COEPS fibres produces
spasticity as mentioned above. For spasticity to develop some
facilitatory pathway to the spinal reflex arc must remain and this
is either the vestibulospinal or reticulospinal tract in man. One
simple version is given here:

(i) Corticospinal tract lesion in the spinal cord—if small
lesion and vestibulospinal tract intact→paraplegia-in-

extension; larger lesion and interrupting the vestibulo-spinal→paraplegia-in-flexion.

This concept is now opposed by some neurologists.

(ii) Extrapyramidal lesions—produce rigidity rather than the spasticity of corticospinal (together with COEPS) tract lesions and affects opposing muscle groups (spasticity affects one or other of the opposing muscle groups, either the flexors or the extensors of the limb), e.g. Parkinsonism.

(iii) Muscular origin—as in myopathic disorders like dystrophia myotonica and myotonia congenita.

Posture

The basic reflex involved in posture is the stretch reflex (Sherrington), seen in its clearest form in the cat when facilitatory influences (from higher centres) upon the stretch reflex are removed, i.e. in decerebrate rigidity. There are various degrees of complexity of reflexes involved in altering posture, these being studied extensively by a pupil of Sherrington, Magnus, who recorded them in his book *Korperstellung*. The various postural reflexes are:

(i) local static ones—originate in the muscles themselves, e.g. the stretch reflex;

(ii) segmental reflexes—arise from the effects of movement of one extremity on the position of the opposite one, e.g. the crossed extensor reflex (noxious stimulus to one leg causes flexion, the flexor reflex, with extension of the opposite limb);

(iii) general static reactions—arise from the actual position of the head in space; receptors in the neck muscles and the labyrinth affect the position of the limbs. In the decerebrate animal, flexion of neck→flexion of forelimbs, etc.

More complex postural reflexes occur in decorticate preparations, e.g. drop blindfolded decorticate cat upside down and it will fall on its paws—a righting reflex (which depends on the labyrinths and neck muscles).

One of the main functions of muscle tone is considered to be the maintenance of posture, and sometimes the posture of the limbs and body are clinically altered due to pathological changes in muscle tone, e.g. hemiplegia, decerebrate rigidity and Parkinsonism.

However the main difficulty with this view is that there may be no disturbance of posture in the presence of abnormal muscle tone (e.g. with the hypotonia of cerebellar disease there is no disturbance of posture, and severe postural deformity in many extrapyramidal diseases occurs when there is hypotonia). This is because the tendon jerks are monosynaptic and lead to synchronous contraction of many muscle fibres, whereas the control of movement at joints is dependent on the rate at which muscles are being moved. It is important to note that consideration of "muscle tone" in patients must take into account the fact that healthy human muscle at rest is electrically silent (e.g. human standing at ease when quadriceps muscle is silent electrically). It is in this area that classical neurophysiology and clinical neurology are difficult to reconcile at the present time.

CEREBRAL CORTEX

Man owes his superiority in the animal world to the enormous development of his cerebral cortex. Attempts have been made for centuries to determine the functional significance of regions of the cerebral cortex in man (back to phrenology), but it is only in the past 100 years that any progress has been made. The clinicians, Broca and Hughlings Jackson, considered that there are motor areas in the brain subserving particular functions (one being for speech) and stimulation of various parts of the

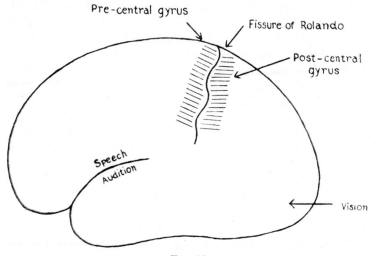

Fig. 19

brain in man and monkeys showed this to be true (Ferrier, de Barenne, and more recently the Canadian neurosurgeon, Penfield). Although there are now considered to be various areas of the cerebral cortex in man which perform specific functions (i.e. "localisation of functions") these are not so discrete physiologically as once thought, although useful for clinical localisation of cortical disease.

Corticospinal (Pyramidal) Tract

The fibres of this tract originate in the cerebral cortex and pass down to spinal cord motor neurones, and many of the fibres originate from cells in the precentral gyrus, the so-called motor area. However, many start from the postcentral gyrus and parietal lobe so the origin of fibres concerned in initiating movement is not as discrete as described in earlier work. Some of the fibres from the cortex do not pass through the pyramids as the pyramidal tract but go to subcortical structures, e.g. the reticular formation, before reaching the spinal motor neurones and are part of the extrapyramidal system (the cortically originating extrapyramidal system, COEPS—see previously). Stimulation of the motor cortex causes movements rather than individual muscle contraction, and the area of cortex representing movements of various areas of the body varies with the delicacy of the movements produced, e.g. large area of motor cortex subserves hand and finger movements. However, the role of COEPS in the execution of skilled movements is greater than once thought and the exact physiological role of the cortical areas subserving movement is under discussion at present.

Clinical.—Precentral tumours or vascular lesions are easy to localise as they cause either stimulation of the region (and consequent Jacksonian epilepsy) or destruction of the region with weakness of the part of the body corresponding to the position of the cortical lesion (e.g. a monoplegia on the opposite side of body). In hemiplegia due to lesions of the internal capsule there is spasticity which cannot be produced in monkeys by lesions in precentral gyrus—so in man spasticity is considered due to damage to the COEPS.

SENSORY CORTEX

The postcentral gyrus contains areas representing sensory impulses from contralateral regions of the body (there is an orderly arrangement of regions represented as there is for the precentral gyrus). Stimulation leads to sensory symptoms in specific body areas but these are not clearly formed (not heat or cold, etc., but rather sensation of movement without any occurring, or tingling). Destruction or ablation reduces the ability to distinguish texture, weight, form.

Clinical.—Irritation of postcentral gyrus causes sensory Jacksonian fits, usually paraesthesiae, whereas destruction (e.g. tumour) leads to sensory loss involving spatial and discriminative aspects of sensation, e.g. tactile discrimination, failure to recognise objects placed in the hand (tactile agnosia).

The parietal cortex lying posteriorly to the postcentral gyrus is concerned with more complex integration of sensations, e.g.:

lesion posterior part left parietal lobe causes disturbance of speech (on its receptive side);

lesions left angular gyrus cause dyslexia and dysgraphia;

lesions right angular gyrus cause disturbance of awareness of the opposite side of the body (a special form of agnosia);

left parieto-occipital area lesion causes visual agnosia (failure to recognise common objects which are clearly seen)

(agnosia means failure of recognition and can be visual, auditory or tactile according to the sensation involved).

PREFRONTAL LOBE

This lies in front of the precentral gyrus and ablation leads to changes in behaviour, e.g. bilateral ablation in monkeys leads to hyperactivity of stereotyped nature at first followed by changes in the memory for recent events. On the basis of this work on monkeys, Moniz introduced the operation of frontal lobotomy for man in 1935 and thus altered disorders characterised by emotional tension (e.g. anxiety neuroses, involutional depression) with reduction of the tension. Depending on the frontal lobe damage produced there is a change in personality (e.g. the famous case of Phineas P. Gage who had a tamping iron through his frontal region and was considered "to be no longer Gage" with regard to his character), e.g. highly distractable, lack of foresight, inability to plan, emotional dullness, even apathy.

These changes are due to complex inter-relations between this area of cortex and the limbic system (the latter is a medial complex of cortex, subcortical nuclei and the tracts which connect them with the hypothalamus and other structures—the limbic system includes the hippocampus, olfactory tubercle, amygdala, cingulate gyrus and connections to thalamus and hypothalamus). The full anatomical and physiological inter-relations are not worked out but in one phase they are concerned with emotion. (See later under Emotion.)

Clinical.—Frontal lobotomy used to be employed for certain psychiatric disorders although drug therapy is now generally preferred. Prefrontal tumours are often hard to localise and they may present with non-specific features such as headaches and generalised convulsions, but a unilateral grasp reflex is suggestive of a frontal lobe lesion. Pressure on neighbouring structures (e.g. Broca's area, olfactory nerve) helps with localisation.

TEMPORAL LOBE

Intimately connects with auditory and visual association areas, with the prefrontal cortex and the limbic system. A small area is concerned with hearing (see later under Hearing). In monkeys part of this lobe is involved in visual discrimination and the comprehension of visual impulses.

Clinical.—Irritating lesions can cause epilepsy with visual and auditory hallucinations (an hallucination is a perception occurring in the absence of an outside stimulus, e.g. hearing a voice when no one is talking) which may also involve the sense of smell: some of these hallucinations may be complex images corresponding to previous events in the patient's life (the "déjà vu" phenomenon). There may be tinnitus (a sensation of noise) with the auditory hallucinations, and with left-sided lesions there may be aphasia (a disorder of the symbolic function of speech, e.g. difficulty naming well-known objects, under-standing speech or writing). Epileptic attacks may be ushered in by unpleasant olfactory sensations ("uncinate epilepsy"). Due to the close proximity of the optic radiation (see under Vision) visual field defects may occur (e.g. homonymous upper quadrantic hemianopia).

OCCIPITAL LOBE

The cortical areas subserving vision lie here and disturbances causing stimulation of this region of the brain produce visual aura, while destruction causes visual field defects (crossed homonymous hemianopia): left occipital lobe lesions may cause visual agnosia.

CORPUS CALLOSUM

As the neocortex has become more evolved it has taken over the prime role of processing and storage of sensory data and the direction of motor response. A system of fibres connecting the neocortical surfaces of the two hemispheres has evolved at the same time, and in higher mammals these fibres are contained in the corpus callosum. Its role is the transmission of information relating to sensory receptive and sensory integrative processes. In primates the corpus callosum is involved in the exchange of information on tactile discrimination learning (training) between the hemispheres, hence, in essence, it is involved in the interhemispheric handling of sensory information (e.g. tactile and visual, and also possibly auditory information).

THE E.E.G. AND EPILEPSY

The cells of the cerebral cortex exhibit rhythmic alterations of electrical potential which can be picked up from the scalp (electroencephalogram). The main wave patterns of the E.E.G. are:

alpha rhythm—8 – 13/sec. (blocked when visual attention involved);

beta rhythm —14 – 60/sec.;

theta rhythm —4 – 7/sec.;

delta rhythm —1 – 3/sec. (an area of cortical damage may be indicated by a localised area of slow delta waves);

abnormal discharges—these are characteristic of epilepsy (which is really a repetitive paroxysmal discharge of abnormal electrical rhythm in some part of the brain).

Clinical types of epilepsy:

(i) petit mal—characteristic wave-and-spike dysrhythmia possibly due to a congenital disorder causing abnormal discharges from the diencephalon (the diencephalon is essentially thalamus + hypothalamus);

(ii) grand mal—various forms of aura (or warning of the attack) precede the actual attack of unconsciousness in which there is tonic spasm of muscles (followed by a clonic phase). The type of aura gives a clue to the origin of the abnormal electrical discharge (due to some "localisation of function" in the cerebral cortex). There are multiple high voltage spikes, widespread and synchronous in both hemispheres of the cortex—possibly due to involvement of some central diencephalic structure;

(iii) temporal lobe epilepsy—important feature is a disturbance of the content of consciousness, e.g. sensory hallucinations or abnormal emotional experiences such as the "déjà vu" phenomenon;

(iv) Jacksonian epilepsy—originates in the precentral motor cortex with clonic movements of regions with the greatest area of representation (thumb, angle of mouth, great toe) followed by spread of this movement throughout body and finally loss of consciousness.

(v) Other forms of epilepsy are variants of above, e.g.:
sudden falling to the ground (akinetic epilepsy);
due to some external stimulus (reflex epilepsy);
persistent clonic movements confined to one part of the body (epilepsia partialis continua);

(vi) myoclonus—a brief, sudden muscular contraction, and the commonest form is that associated with epilepsy.

Consciousness

The E.E.G. of the alert animal and the sleeping animal differ and this change can be produced by electrical stimulation of the reticular formation (*reticular formation*—those areas of the brain stem made up of diffuse aggregations of cells of different types + intermingling fibres but excluding circumscribed groups of cells like the red nucleus, the facial nucleus, etc.). Sensory afferent impulses feed into the reticular formation which, in turn, changes the E.E.G. pattern (i.e. affects the cortical neurones) presumably due to desynchronisation of cortical cellular activity. Hence the central reticular formation is the anatomical basis of an alerting system.

Loss of consciousness is considered due to interference with the activity of the central reticular formation.

Clinical.—*Coma* is a prolonged state of unconsciousness (due to interference with reticular formation function) and may be produced by:

(i) Cerebral vascular lesions, e.g. massive subarachnoid haemorrhage; large intracerebral haemorrhage; large area of oedema due to infarction of central reticular formation (e.g. thrombosis of basilar artery).

(ii) Space-occupying lesions, e.g. intracranial tumour or abscess; subdural haematoma.

(iii) Head injury.

(iv) Meningitis and encephalitis.

(v) Drugs, e.g. aspirin, barbiturates, morphine, alcohol.

(vi) Metabolic disorders, e.g. uraemia, diabetic ketosis, hypoglycaemia, hepatic dysfunction.

(vii) Endocrine disorders, e.g. myxoedema, hypopituitarism, suprarenal cortical failure.

(viii) CO or CO_2 intoxication.

(ix) Epilepsy.

THE EYE

Refraction

An image of the external environment is formed on the retina by the lens of the eye. The focal length of the lens can be changed by the ciliary muscle which alters the curvature of the lens and this is known as *accommodation* (when the ciliary muscle is relaxed the lens is flattened). The image may be formed in front of the retina—*myopia* (treated by concave lens for distant vision) or formed behind the retina—*hyperopia* (use converging lenses) or there may be a reduced ability to accommodate — *presbyopia* — or the corneal surface may not be spherical—*astigmatism*.

The pupil.—The iris forms an excellent diaphragm to alter the amount of light falling on the retina (constriction increases depth of focus of lens and helps form clear image—iris constricts in conjunction with accommodation and convergence for near vision). The pupil size is changed by the muscles of the iris, the sphincter and dilator muscles. The eye itself is moved by the external muscles supplied by the 3rd, 4th and 6th cranial nerves. Both the smooth intrinsic and striate extrinsic muscles of the eye are controlled by a group of nuclei in the midbrain.

An increase in light intensity causes the pupil to constrict and vice versa, and the innervation of the pupil is:

```
sympathetic fibres from brain stem ──► Ist thoracic ──► stellate ──► cervical ──► enter skull
                                        spinal cord     ganglion    sympathetic   with
                                        segment                     trunk         internal
                                                                                  carotid
                                                                                  artery
                                                                                    │
                                                                                    ▼
                                                         dilatation of ◄────── eye
                                                         pupil

III nerve nucleus ──► enter III ──► ciliary ganglion ──► circular muscle ──► irido-constrictor
                      cranial                            of eye              muscles
                      nerve
```

Reaction of pupil to light—afferent side of reflex are visual pathways to superior colliculus and then to iridoconstrictor part of 3rd nerve nucleus.

Clinical.—Abnormal pupil:

(i) Argyll Robertson pupil—reacts on accommodation normally, but not to light (due to neurosyphilis) (for explanation see under The Reflex Arc earlier).

(ii) Holmes–Adie syndrome—females: markedly reduced reaction to light and abnormally slow constriction of pupil on convergence often associated with decreased tendon jerks.

(iii) Hutchinsonian pupil—widely dilated and unreactive due to increased intracranial pressure and in cardiac arrest (due to hypoxia of III nerve nucleus).

(iv) Horner's syndrome—small pupil and ptosis of the upper lid due to interference with the sympathetic nerve supply to the eye.

(v) Optic nerve damage—direct reflexes absent but consensual reflexes brisk; commonest causes are retrobulbar neuritis and optic nerve compression.

Intraocular Fluid

The pressure inside the eye is normally $20 - 25$ mm.Hg resulting from a balance between the formation (chiefly from the blood by the ciliary body) of intraocular fluid and its escape (by leakage into the canal of Schlemm and thence into the intrascleral veins). Interference with drainage causes increased intraocular pressure, *glaucoma*, which can damage vision.

The Fundus

One important feature of the eye is that it is the only region of the body in which blood vessels can be examined directly (with an ophthalmoscope) and also the head of the optic nerve can be visualised directly.

Clinical features determined from examination of the fundus:

(a) Blood vessels—these may be changed by:

  hypertension—compression of veins by arteries, also leak of blood (haemorrhage) or presence of oedema fluid in nerve fibres (exudates);

  atherosclerosis—narrowing and irregularity of the lumen of the arteries of the retina;

  diabetes (where minute swellings, or micro-aneurysms, occur);

  renal disease.

(b) The optic nerve—as this is surrounded by the cerebro-spinal fluid, examination of the optic disc can be used to detect increase in intracranial pressure which causes elimination of the normal physiological optic cup as the nerve head becomes swollen (papilloedema):

Papilloedema may be due to:

  (i) increased intracranial pressure (due to hypertension, intracranial tumour, brain abscess);

 (ii) inflammatory lesion of the optic nerve (optic neuritis);

(iii) thrombosis of central vein of retina.

Optic atrophy.—Atrophy of the optic nerve (disc): caused by:

  (i) disseminated sclerosis;

 (ii) neurosyphilis;

(iii) obstruction of central artery of retina;

(iv) pressure on the optic nerve by tumour or increased intraocular pressure (glaucoma);

 (v) continued increased intracranial pressure (i.e. end result of papilloedema);

(vi) toxic substances, e.g. tobacco, methyl alcohol, trypars-amide, etc.;

(vii) certain degenerative diseases of the nervous system, e.g. familial spastic paraplegia, etc.

Vision.—There are two end organs in the eye:

(*a*) rods for night vision, low threshold, no colour vision, poor perception of detail;

(*b*) cones for colour vision, fovea has only cones, able to determine fine detail.

The rods contain the pigment, visual purple (rhodopsin) which is bleached by light and this photochemical process produces a nerve impulse which passes down the optic nerve.

Light—rhodopsin—excitatory decomposition product

—nerve impulse

Wald established the broad outlines of the photochemistry of the visual cycle:

$$\text{Rhodopsin (a conjugated protein)} \underset{\text{dark}}{\overset{\text{light}}{\rightleftharpoons}} \text{retinene (a pigment + protein group)}$$

Rhodopsin itself is produced slowly from vitamin A.

Colour vision is possible because of three pigments in the cones (probably in three separate types of cone) sensitive to red, green and blue light and they are therefore capable of detecting any colour (the Young–Helmholtz theory). A violet-sensitive substance, iodopsin, has been isolated by Wald, and recently a blue receptor has been demonstrated.

Colour blindness may be:

(i) acquired (variety of retinal, systemic and toxic disorders); difficulty with blue and yellow vision is usually acquired;

(ii) congenital because of an inherited lack of some mechanism vital to colour vision, e.g. red-green blindness (male sex-linked inheritance), total colour blindness (inherited as a simple recessive trait).

Visual fields.—The visual field of an eye is the extent of the external world which can be seen with the eye looking fixedly forward. The pathway for vision is as follows:

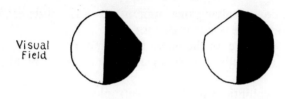

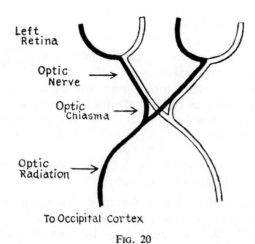

Fig. 20

Central visual pathways:

Ganglion cells of ──→ Nerve fibres ──→ Optic chiasma ──→ lateral geniculate body
inner layer of   (the optic   (synapse here)
retina   nerve)

Occipital lobe

pretectal region close to
superior colliculus
(constitute afferent limb
of pupillary reflexes to
light)

Fibres from the macula of the retina (cones only here) tend to finish in a discrete area in the posterior part of the calcarine fissure of the occiptal lobe, and this area may be spared when ischaemia affects the occipital cortex because it receives a double blood supply (causes "tunnel vision").

Clinical.—Lesions of the optic tract in various parts cause the following visual defects:

(i) lesion involving one optic nerve → visual defect limited to the eye concerned, e.g.:

    pressure on the nerve by a tumour;

    retrobulbar neuritis leading to a central blind area or scotoma;

    syphilitic primary optic atrophy;

    advanced papilloedema;

(ii) lesion of optic chiasma, e.g. pituitary tumour causes bitemporal hemianopia;

(iii) lesion of one optic tract

(iv) lesion of optic radiation   } causes crossed homonymous hemianopia;

(v) lesion of visual cortex, e.g. thrombosis posterior cerebral artery

(vi) lesion of visual cortex with sparing of the area of occipital cortex concerned with macular vision (because of a dual blood supply to this area) causes telescopic or tunnel vision.

Nystagmus.—Disturbance of ocular posture characterized by rhythmical oscillation of the eyes:

(i) retinal origin—due to defective vision, e.g. amblyopia early in life, persistent dim light as in miner's nystagmus;

(ii) disorders of labyrinth—usually rotatory, e.g. acute lesions of internal ear;

(iii) due to central lesions—especially of brain stem and cerebellum, e.g. disseminated sclerosis, but also in hereditary ataxia, syringomyelia, tumours and vascular lesions of brain stem and cerebellum;

(iv) congenital.

THE EAR

The ear subserves two sensory modalities, namely hearing and equilibration.

Hearing

The auditory system is composed of the following parts:

(*a*) the outer ear;

(*b*) middle ear;

(*c*) cochlea;

(*d*) auditory nerve and pathways to central neural structures.

(a) and (b) are concerned in the transmission of sound waves from the external environment to the cochlea where these waves are transformed into nerve impulses which pass down the auditory nerve (VIIIth cranial nerve). Sound waves impinging on the tympanic membrane move it and this movement is transmitted through the three bony ossicles to the membrane sealing the oval window and causes compression of the fluid in the cochlea. Compression of the fluid in the cochlea moves the basilar membrane stimulating the organ of Corti (the hair cells of the organ of Corti are distorted, the nerve endings of the cochlea branch of VIIIth nerve are stimulated and impulses pass down this nerve to central structures).

Békésy has concluded that the "place" and "frequency" theories of the older physiology textbooks are, in fact, closely related. The basilar membrane responds to the pressure waves which reach it via the oval window and are transmitted through the fluid of the inner ear. These waves travel through the basilar membrane, and low frequencies displace the entire membrane in a whiplike fashion while high frequencies damp out a short distance from the stapes (hence *high* tones are represented at the *base* of the cochlea and low tones throughout the cochlea but with maximum effectiveness near the apex)—this is known as the *travelling wave theory of Békésy*.

CENTRAL AUDITORY PATHWAYS

The VIIIth nerve fibres synapse in the dorsal and ventral cochlea nuclei which connect with the superior olivary complex (fibres from there go to motor nuclei in brain stem and reticular formation and also to the cerebellum) and then to the inferior colliculus (for auditory reflexes rather than hearing) and the medial geniculate body and thence to the cortical auditory centre in the temporal lobe (where there is bilateral representation for hearing).

Deafness

Conduction deafness—interference with passage of sound waves to the organ of hearing, the cochlea:

  (a) external ear blockage, e.g. by wax;
  (b) middle ear, e.g. adhesions of ossicles to bony walls or growth of new bone that binds the stapes (otosclerosis); otitis media.

Nerve (or perceptive) deafness—defect lies in cochlea or nerve pathways from it:

(c) damage to sensory cells of organ of Corti, e.g. boiler-makers' deafness, Ménière's syndrome;

(d) lesion of auditory (VIIIth) nerve, e.g. tumour in cerebello-pontine angle, especially an acoustic neuroma;

(e) lesions in temporal lobe do not cause deafness unless bilateral.

Two tests are used to distinguish middle ear from nerve deafness:

Weber's test—tuning fork to mid-forehead:
normal ears—sound appears in midline;
conductive deafness—localised in affected (or deafer) ear;
nerve deafness—localised in normal ear.
Rinne's test is based on similar principles.

Tinnitus is a sensation of noise caused by abnormal excitation of the cochlea, VIIIth nerve or its pathways to the cerebral cortex. May originate in:

(i) internal ear (commonest cause): often associated with deafness and sometimes vertigo, e.g. Ménière's syndrome; drugs, e.g. streptomycin, quinine, salicylates; circulatory disorders;

(ii) VIIIth nerve, e.g. acoustic neuroma (the auditory nuclei and ascending pathways are rarely affected);

(iii) auditory cortex, e.g. tumour here can cause tinnitus.

Equilibration

The labyrinth consists of the semicircular canals, utricle and saccule. The semicircular canals lie at right angles to one another and each contains a ridge, the crista, on which are hair-like processes closely related to the vestibular fibres of VIIIth nerve—changes in rotational movement cause a distortion of these processes by movement of the fluid (endolymph) in the semicircular canals. Hence these end-organs detect any change in the rate of movement of the head in space (angular accelera-tion or deceleration) while the utricle detects the static position of the head and linear acceleration (their end-organs have small particles in them called otoliths which change position in response to tilting and linear acceleration) (the function of the saccule is not clearly defined but may detect slow vibrational stimuli rather than being an essential part of the vestibular apparatus).

The vestibular fibres enter the pons and end in the vestibular nuclei or run directly to the cerebellum. Fibres from the vestibular nerve run up to the temporal lobe or down in the vestibulospinal tracts to influence spinal motor neurones. The labyrinths are, therefore, concerned with the position and movement of the body in space.

Clinical.—Vertigo is an awareness of disordered orientation of the body in space due to the following causes:

(i) disturbance of sensory end-organ. Disturbance of function of the labyrinth is by far the commonest cause (aural vertigo) due to unaccustomed stimuli acting on normal labyrinths (e.g. motion sickness) and Ménière's syndrome (recurrent aural vertigo, vomiting, tinnitus, increasing deafness);

(ii) afferent paths, e.g.:
epidemic vertigo probably due to vestibular neuronitis (? virus infection);
central lesions affecting vestibular nerve, their connections or cerebellum;
disseminated sclerosis, syringomyelia, neoplastic lesions, vascular (especially occlusion of the posterior inferior cerebellar artery);

(iii) central mechanism, e.g.:
cortical origin in migraine;
"giddiness" common complaint in anxiety neurosis.

CEREBELLUM

This can influence motor neurones only indirectly (through connections with motor systems of brain stem and the cerebral cortex), and its chief function is the regulation of posture, muscle tone and movement (especially voluntary skilled movements). Consistent with this complex function there is a rich supply of afferent and efferent connections.

Afferent input from proprioceptors

vestibular system
visual and auditory sensory systems
cerebral cortex.

Efferent output to cerebral cortex

brain stem structures (which give rise to descending pathways).

Functions

Equilibration.—Especially, but not only, the flocculonodular lobe. The stretch reflex supplies the information essential for posture, but this basic reflex must be controlled, and equilibration is one part of this control (in which the vestibular system is important) but vision and proprioception are also involved. Standing involves three main sensory inputs to the cerebellum (vestibular, proprioceptive, visual) and the cerebellum then exerts control over the body musculature.

Tone.—The stretch reflex is regulated by higher centres (vestibular nuclei and brain stem reticular system) and the cerebellum also helps control muscle tone.

Control of voluntary movements.—Defects in cerebellar control show as errors in rate, range, force and direction of voluntary movements (ataxia) and coarse irregular oscillations especially at the termination of movement (intention tremor).

CLINICAL FEATURES

Tone.—Cerebellar disease may cause hypotonia (therefore cerebellar impulses are facilitatory to the stretch reflex).

Voluntary movement.—Cerebellar deficiency causes a disturbance of the mechanism by which posture and movement are normally regulated, and tremor develops if an attempt is made to maintain limb in a fixed posture and also on movement (increasing tremor as object approached—intention tremor). Nystagmus is really tremor in attempt to keep the eyes fixed in one position and is usually present in cerebellar disease, e.g. disseminated sclerosis is commonest cause of nystagmus.

Gait.—Altered due to difficulty with equilibration (walk on a broad base).

These disorders all give rise to various degrees of cerebellar deficiency:

disseminated sclerosis;
medulloblastoma or astrocytoma in cerebellum in children;
degenerative lesion of cerebellum as in Friedreich's ataxia;

progressive cerebellar degeneration of unknown cause in middle life or due to carcinoma;

thrombosis posterior inferior cerebellar artery.

BASAL GANGLIA

Basal ganglia are involved in the control of movement and posture and include all subcortical motor nuclei of the forebrain including the caudate nucleus, putamen and globus pallidus: they discharge to the following structures:

subthalamic nucleus of Luys;

substantia nigra;

red nucleus;

reticular formation in the brain stem.

Sometimes all the above are included in the term "basal ganglia". There are complex pathways between the various parts of the basal ganglia and the motor cortex but essentially the basal ganglia moderate movements, and most of the information on their function has come from the results of human disease.

Clinical.—The *extrapyramidal syndromes* are disorders which result from lesions involving parts of the brain other than corticospinal pathways, which are concerned with movement (especially the basal ganglia and connections). The extra-pyramidal syndromes include:

(i) The Parkinsonian syndrome (due to idiopathic causes, encephalitis, carbon monoxide, manganese, reserpine, chlorpromazine) with the immobile face, involuntary tremor and rigidity and disorder of volitional movement (micrographia, festinating gait, etc.).

Sometimes due to degeneration of the substantia nigra and possibly consequent overactivity of the globus pallidus. The syndrome can sometimes be relieved by surgical lesions of the globus pallidus and of ventral nucleus of the thalamus.

(ii) Hepatolenticular degeneration (Wilson's disease) — familial degeneration of corpus striatum with cirrhosis of the liver due to deficient plasma caeruloplasmin (which carries copper in the blood) with deposition of copper in these tissues: increased muscular rigidity and tremor.

(iii) Chorea—involuntary movements of quasi-purposive nature due to:

rheumatic fever (Sydenham's chorea);

hereditary degeneration corpus striatum (and fore-brain)—Huntingdon's chorea;

damage to basal ganglia due to excess blood bilirubin in the jaundiced newborn—kernicterus;

hemiballismus—lesion involving opposite subthalamic nucleus of Luys causing violent choreiform movements.

(iv) Athetosis—slow, coarse, writhing movements either bilateral (usually congenital and with or without pyramidal tract lesions—if with them regarded as a form of congenital diplegia) or unilateral (associated with infantile hemiplegia). Although the specific nature of the lesion is not clear, a surgical lesion of globus pallidus may be beneficial (as for (i) above).

THE AUTONOMIC NERVOUS SYSTEM

Like the somatic nervous system this is based on the reflex arc:

VISCERAL RECEPTORS —(Afferent Impulses)→ CENTRAL NERVOUS SYSTEM (integrated at various levels) —(Efferent Impulses)→ VISCERAL EFFECTORS (e.g. smooth muscle of blood vessels, glands, etc.)

There are two main anatomical divisions, the sympathetic and parasympathetic nervous systems.

Sympathetic nervous system.—The cells of origin lie in the intermediolateral column of spinal cord from C8 to L2 – 3 spinal segments and the axons of those cells leave the spinal cord by the corresponding anterior nerve roots and synapse with nerve cells in outlying ganglia. Axons arise from nerve cells in the ganglia (non-medullated, postganglionic) and go to muscle cells or glands (a few fibres do not synapse in the ganglia of the sympathetic chain but much closer to the effector organ as illustrated). There are higher controlling centres over this system from the cerebral cortex, hypothalamus and medulla.

Sympathetic fibres in the head and neck go to blood vessels, sweat glands, pilomotor muscles in head and neck, and to salivary glands and dilator muscles of pupil. Those to the thoracic viscera go to the heart, lungs and oesophagus where they form plexuses with branches from the vagus nerve (Xth cranial nerve). The abdominal and pelvic visceral sections of the sympathetic nervous system go to nearly all abdominal organs and rich plexuses of fibres are formed in relation to the aorta and its branches.

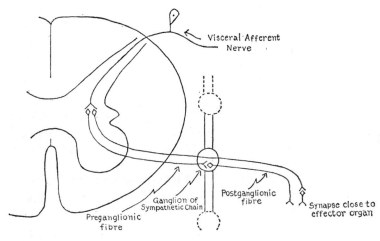

FIG. 21

Parasympathetic nervous system.—This more scattered system has cell stations for its fibres in:

(i) the *midbrain*—Edinger–Westphal nucleus of IIIrd cranial nerve (which gives rise to iridoconstrictor fibres);

(ii) *medulla*—superior salivary nucleus supplying the salivary and lacrymal glands and fauces and pharynx;
dorsal nucleus of vagus—fibres go to thoracic and abdominal viscera (the ganglion cells of the post-ganglionic fibres usually lie within the organs innervated);

(iii) *sacral*—cell stations in S2–4 part of spinal cord supplying fibres to descending colon, rectum and bladder.

Afferent impulses from the viscera probably go by corresponding nerve fibres but the anatomical picture here is less clear.

Functions of the Autonomic Nervous System

It innervates smooth muscle, cardiac muscle and glands and is concerned with regulating the vegetative functions of the body and with emergency mechanisms concerned with fighting, exercise, etc. (compare with the somatic nerves which innervate voluntary muscle and adjust organism in relation to the external environment). More specifically these functions are concerned with the activity of:

> cardiac muscle,
> smooth muscle,
> digestive glands,
> sweat glands,
> adrenal medulla.

Most effector organs of the autonomic nervous system are innervated by both sympathetic and parasympathetic nerves, e.g.:

> heart—rate of beating reduced by vagus and increased by sympathetic nerves;
> intestine—movement inhibited by sympathetic and increased by parasympathetic stimulation.

When the sympathetic chains are removed from an animal it can live satisfactorily only in a sheltered environment and:

> cannot do hard exercise;
> reactions to cold environment fail;
> less able to withstand haemorrhage than a normal animal.

The parasympathetic effects are more localised in character. Some specific examples of the effect of the autonomic nervous system are given below:

Organ supplied	Sympathetic	Para-sympathetic
Pupil (ciliary muscle)	Dilated	Constricted
Parotid gland	No secretion	Profuse watery secretion
Lungs (bronchial muscle)	Relaxed	Constricted
Blood vessels (skin)	Constricted	—
Heart rate	Increased	Decreased
Intestinal motility	Decreased	Increased
Adrenal medulla (preganglionic fibres)	Secretion of adrenaline and noradrenaline	—

Humoral Transmission of Nerve Impulses

The substance acetylcholine is released at the terminations of all nerves with the *only exception* of most sympathetic postganglionic fibres (i.e. after the initial synapse which separates a postganglionic fibre from the preganglionic sympathetic fibre which is the axon of the neurone whose cell station lies in the intermediolateral column of the spinal cord). Acetylcholine released by the nerve ending (i.e. cholinergic nerve) diffuses across the synapse or neuromuscular junction to depolarise the postsynaptic membrane (may be a postganglionic fibre or skeletal muscle membrane or a gland or other effector organ).

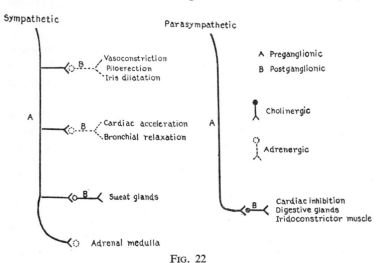

FIG. 22

At the terminations of most postganglionic sympathetic fibres noradrenaline is released (i.e. adrenergic fibres), the exception being sympathetic postganglionic fibres to sweat glands and blood vessels of skeletal muscle at which acetylcholine is released (i.e. sympathetic postganglionic cholinergic fibres). The details are summarised in Fig. 22.

APPLIED PHARMACOLOGICAL ASPECTS OF HUMORAL TRANSMISSION

Actylcholine is synthesised by choline acetylase in the nerve fibres and after its release it is destroyed by hydrolysis by the enzyme cholinesterase (this enzyme is inhibited by physostigmine, whose other name is eserine, and neostigmine, di-isopropylfluorophosphate, DFP, and the "nerve gases"; this leads to the persistence of secreted acetylcholine which blocks nerve transmission).

Acetylcholine released at the neuromuscular junction to skeletal muscle causes muscle contraction—the access of acetylcholine to the motor end-plate is blocked by curare and gallamine ("Flaxedil") leading to paralysis of voluntary movement. The drugs succinylcholine and decamethonium also combine with receptor sites on the motor end-plate leading to persistent depolarisation of the muscle membrane and paralysis of the muscle (see Chapter XI). These drugs are used for relaxation of skeletal muscle in anaesthesia to render the surgeon's task easier. Many drugs block the stimulation of effector cells (other than skeletal muscle) by acetylcholine, e.g. atropine, scopolamine (a chemical isomer of atropine) and are also used in anaesthesia to prevent excess mucus production by the glands of the bronchial mucosa.

The smooth muscle of many blood vessels is innervated by sympathetic adrenergic postganglionic fibres and is responsible for the tone or vasoconstriction usually present (except blood vessels to skeletal muscles and sweat glands). As the blood pressure of an individual is the resultant of cardiac output and the resistance against which the blood is ejected, it can be understood how blood pressure can be changed by altering either cardiac output or vasoconstrictor tone (see Chapter III). In benign essential hypertension cardiac output is normal but there is an abnormal degree of vasoconstrictor tone and this can be reduced by therapy. Some years ago this therapy was aimed at blocking transmission between pre- and postganglionic sympathetic fibres (using "ganglion-blockers" such as hexamethonium, mecamylamine), but this caused rather widespread and distressing side-effects; more recently drugs which block the action of postganglionic fibres have come into prominence and these have fewer side-effects—the most useful nowadays are:

    (i) guanethidine—interferes with the uptake and release of noradrenaline from nerve endings;

    (ii) methyldopa—metabolised to α-methyl noradrenaline which is only a weak transmitter at sympathetic nerve endings;

(iii) reserpine—depletes tissue stores of noradrenaline: also has a central action.

Catecholamine Metabolism

Adrenaline and noradrenaline are synthesised from phenylalanine via tyrosine and dihydroxyphenylalanine (DOPA), and are degraded to 3-methoxy, 4-hydroxy mandelic acid (synonym is Vanil mandelic acid or VMA) and conjugates of metanephrine and normetanephrine. When excess catecholamines are produced as in phaeochromocytoma (see Chapter II) there is an increase in urinary VMA excretion.

Higher Control of the Autonomic Nervous System

There are higher centres for the control of the autonomic nervous system, e.g. medullary centres, hypothalamus.

Medullary centres.—These are used to control the blood pressure via the cardioregulatory and vasomotor centres in the medulla (former changes heart rate and stroke volume while latter alters peripheral resistance) (see Chapter III).

Hypothalamus.—This is responsible for the following functions:

(i) *Regulation of body temperature.*—A destructive lesion in the ventral hypothalamus renders an animal incapable of regulating its temperature in a hot environment and may cause hyperthermia (because no sweating or cutaneous vasodilatation occurs). Clinically this is seen in anterior hypothalamic tumours and infarcts. A lesion in the caudal hypothalamus impairs the animal's ability to maintain normal body temperature in a cold environment because of defective cutaneous vasoconstriction, shivering and adrenaline secretion.

There are two co-ordinated thermoregulatory centres in the hypothalamus (which is really a *thermostat* with information obtained from cutaneous thermoreceptors and central thermoreceptors in the hypothalamus itself). The complex activities involved in maintaining body temperature involve the autonomic nervous system which is under the control of the hypothalamus for this purpose.

(ii) *Water balance.*—There are osmoreceptors in the hypothalamus (see Antidiuretic Hormone—Chapter II) and these are involved in regulating water excretion (see Chapter IX). Possibly it also has a function in regulating water intake.

(iii) *Oxytocin release.*—Role unclear.

(iv) *Regulation of adenohypophyseal function.*—Hypothalamic cells secrete chemicals into a portal system which carries them to the sinusoids of the adenohypophysis and regulates the release of hormones from the latter. The hypothalamus is known to produce a corticotrophin releasing factor (CRF), and probably other "releasing factors" regulating the release of thyroid-stimulating hormone, growth hormone and the gonadotropic hormones from the anterior pituitary (hence influencing a great variety of the vegetative functions of the body— see Chapter II).

(v) *Regulation of food intake.*—Damage to parts of hypo-thalamus can produce polyphagia and obesity, or conversely anorexia: this suggests that hypothalamus may act as a feeding centre.

(vi) *Gastric acid secretion.*—The hypothalamus may have a role here: clinically of importance in relation to emotional stress and peptic ulcers.

(vii) *Cardiovascular regulation.*—Electrical stimulation of certain areas of the hypothalamus can produce changes in heart rate and blood pressure but these really represent isolated fragments of a total behavioural pattern such as anger or fear (or the effects of exercise). Also can regulate the capacity of the system venous reservoir and when damaged (as by subarachnoid haemorrhage) can cause the explosive onset of pulmonary oedema.

Emotion.—A way of feeling or acting which can be broken down into three component phases:

(i) cognition—perception and evaluation of the situation and relation to previous experiences;

(ii) expression—somatic and autonomic activities;

(iii) experience—the subjective aspects of emotion (i.e. what one feels when emotional) such as excitement.

There is a large autonomic response to cognitive functions, e.g. cardiac acceleration doing mental arithmetic, and the presence of a hypothalamus alters the reaction to a noxious stimulus to "sham rage" (violent autonomic responses) from an emotional vegetable when the hypothalamus is removed. It appears that the neural mechanisms for the basic elements of sexual behaviour and rage are located in the hypothalamus. Stimulation of hypothalamus can cause flight or rage pattern, e.g. pupillary dilatation, pilo-erection, growling, etc., in experimental animals and these are patterns of behaviour involving integrated visceral and somatic responses of the body as a whole.

The hypothalamus is connected to the limbic system (see above under Prefrontal Lobe) and this functional unit (together with ascending and descending pathways) is concerned in the visceral and somatic aspects of emotion, but also probably in the cognitive and other subjective aspects of emotion as well.

CEREBROSPINAL FLUID

The *meninges* (or coverings) of the brain are:

 (i) dura mater—tough, closely applied to cranium: provides two main supports for brain (falx, tentorium);
 (ii) arachnoid—closely applied to dura but a potential space (subdural space) exists between the two;
 (iii) pia mater—applied directly to brain surface but potential space between it and arachnoid (subarachnoid space).

Cerebrospinal fluid is formed by the choroid plexuses (the epithelium of which acts as glandular tissue) in all ventricles, especially the lateral ventricles, and it circulates as follows:

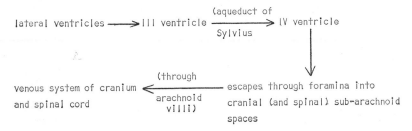

Composition.—Different from plasma due to *active* secretion by choroid plexuses (involves active transport of Na^+ and Cl' and the epithelium of the choroid plexuses can secrete against a pressure gradient and cause a rise in intracranial pressure). The total volume of the cerebrospinal fluid is about 120 ml. There is also a physiological barrier between plasma and C.S.F. which prevents certain substances in the blood entering the C.S.F. (the blood-brain barrier). Normal C.S.F. pressure (lateral position) is 60 – 150 mm. fluid.

Protein: 15 – 40 mg./100 ml. (moderate increase in inflammatory diseases of nervous tissue and meninges; marked rise in obstruction of spinal subarachnoid space and polyneuritis).

Glucose: 50 – 80 mg./100 ml. (reduced in meningitis).

Chloride: 725 – 750 mg/100 ml. (greatly reduced in tuberculous meningitis).

Occasional white cell (<3/cu. mm.)—increased by bacterial infections (especially polymorphonuclear leucocytes) and viral infections (especially mononuclear cells).

Clinical.—Increased intracranial pressure may be due to:

intracranial tumour and haemorrhage,
hypertensive encephalopathy,
benign intracranial hypertension,
meningitis and encephalitis,
hydrocephalus.

Chapter XI

MUSCLE

THE function of muscle is to contract and either move bones in respect to one another (*skeletal* muscle) or exert pressure on the fluid contents of hollow viscera (*cardiac* and *visceral* smooth muscle). This contraction is controlled by the central nervous system, either reflexly or voluntarily, in the case of skeletal muscle, while smooth muscle and cardiac muscle have an inherent rhythmicity of their own which is, in turn, regulated by nervous activity.

Skeletal muscle has been much more extensively studied than smooth muscle and most of this chapter will be concerned with a study of its action. Skeletal muscle is the means by which an organism reacts to its external environment, and it is now possible to relate structure to mechanism of contraction on the basis of the sliding filament model of Huxley.

Structure and Molecular Basis of Contraction

Each muscle consists of many muscle fibres banded together by connective tissue, and each muscle fibre consists of numerous myofibrils embedded in a structureless medium, the sarcoplasm, and bounded by a cell membrane (the sarcolemma). Different refractile and staining properties give muscle a banded appearance, the optically dense or dark bands under the microscope are called A (anisotropic bands which are electron-dense in the electron microscope) while the lighter ones are the I bands (isotropic). The I-band is crossed by the Z-line, a membrane dividing the muscle fibre transversely (the muscle unit, or sarcomere, is the region between two successive Z-bands). Mitochondria, present near the myofibrils, contain the enzymes for the tricarboxylic acid cycle (see Chapter I), whereas glyco-lytic activity lies in non-particulate matter in the sarcoplasm.

Each myofibril consists of numerous minute filaments (myofilaments), some being thick and others thin, and they have been shown by H. E. Huxley to be arranged as shown:

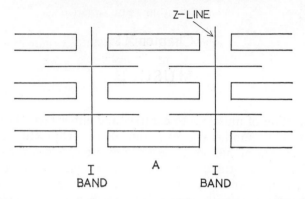

When a muscle shortens the thin filaments (composed of actin) slide over the thick ones (of myosin mainly) by the creation and dissolution of molecular "bridges" between the two types of myofilament. Actin and myosin can be obtained separately, and when mixed they can be spun into a filament which will contract on the addition of adenosine triphosphate (ATP). Myosin is an enzyme which catalyses the hydrolysis of ATP (i.e. it is an ATP-ase and is activated by Ca^{++} and inhibited by Mg^{++}):

$$ATP \xrightarrow[\text{(myosin)}]{} ADP + phosphate$$

The ATP is the source of energy for contraction while Ca ions control the contraction. ATP is probably directly involved in the formation of bridges between the thick and thin filaments. Shortening of the bridge could then bring ATP into the immediate vicinity of the ATP-ase, cause hydrolysis of ATP and break the bridge. There is an extensive membranous tubular structure in the cytoplasm, the *sarcoplasmic reticulum*, which couples the depolarisation of the muscle cell membrane (the sarcolemma) to the contractile machinery. The mechanism of this excitation-contraction coupling is as shown on page 185.

Depolarisation of the sarcolemma is by local circuit currents (see Chapter X) produced by depolarisation at a specialised junction between the motor nerve and the muscle fibre, the motor end-plate. The terminal portions of the motor nerve axon release acetylcholine which diffuses to the muscle motor end-plate and depolarises it (i.e. produces a reversible change in membrane permeability to Na^+ and K^+ ions and hence a change

Depolarisation of the cell membrane
↓
Depolarisation of the part of the sarcoplasmic reticulum directly connected to the cell membrane
↓
Release of Ca^{++} from sarcoplasmic reticulum
↓
Diffuses short distance to region of overlap of thick and thin filaments
↓
Activates myosin and energy produced
↓
Myofilaments slide over one another (i.e. tension generating reaction)
↓
TENSION

in the voltage across the membrane); when the electrical potential produced reaches a threshold value, a wave of depolarisation is propagated over the muscle membrane. The acetylcholine is destroyed by hydrolysis:

Acetylcholine ————→ Inactivation of acetylcholine
(cholinesterase)

The energy for muscle contraction comes from the hydrolysis of the high-energy terminal phosphate group of ATP. The concentration of ATP is maintained by creatine phosphate (CP) in the muscle.

Role of Calcium

Injection of Ca^{++} into an intact muscle causes local contraction and reducing the Ca^{++} concentration causes relaxation. The findings suggest that the contractile activity of myofibrils is controlled by variations in sarcoplasmic calcium concentration; possibly the excitation-contraction coupling mechanism releases calcium to induce contraction, and some mechanism then takes this up to produce relaxation of muscle. The release of calcium may occur near the transverse tubule of the sarcoplasmic reticulum.

Drugs acting at Neuromuscular Junction

Curare and gallamine block the access of acetylcholine to the motor end-plate by combining with receptors on the motor end-plate and preventing the action of acetylcholine. Decamethonium and succinylcholine act like acetylcholine by depolarising the motor end-plate but they are more resistant to the action of cholinesterase than is acetylcholine. The effect of both of these groups of agents is to block neuromuscular transmission and paralyse skeletal muscle. Anticholinesterases (e.g. "nerve gas", certain organic phosphorus pesticides) prevent the action of cholinesterase and hence prevent the destruction of acetylcholine and produce prolonged depolarisation of the motor end-plate (and ultimately paralysis of the muscle); their effect may be reversed by specific cholinesterase activators (oximes which break attachment between the anticholinesterase and cholinesterase) or partly by atropine. Atropine (which renders tissues less sensitive to acetylcholine) appears to prevent death from "nerve gas" in man by preventing depression of the medullary respiratory centre. As acetylcholine is liberated at the ends of nerves to smooth muscle and all autonomic nerve synapses, the above drugs have widespread effects in the body other than on skeletal muscle.

Mechanical Effects

The force developed by a contracting muscle (when all its fibres are stimulated) is related to the initial length at the time of stimulation.

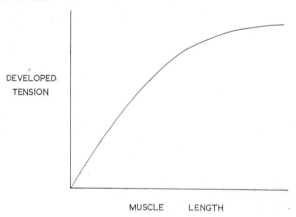

This length-tension relationship is a fundamental property of contracting muscle (a special development of this is seen in Starling's Law of the Heart; see Chapter III). There is a striking correlation between relative overlap of thick and thin filaments at various sarcomere lengths and the length-tension diagram.

The total amount of tension that a muscle can exert under optimal conditions is a function of the total number of fibres and the number of myofilaments per fibre.

CLINICAL DISORDERS OF MUSCLE CONTRACTION

Disease attacks five points in the motor unit (motor unit = single motor neurone, its axon and the group of muscle fibres innervated by it):

(i) *Destruction of cell body*, e.g. acute poliomyelitis.

(ii) *Destruction of nerve axon*, e.g. peripheral nerve injury. Both (i) and (ii) cause a flaccid muscle paralysis with muscle degeneration (causing fibrillation and fasciculation) and reduced or absent tendon reflexes.

(iii) *Neuromuscular junction*, e.g. myasthenia gravis, curare. In myasthenia there is an abnormal response of the motor end-plate to acetylcholine and extreme fatiguability, especially of the facial muscles, is produced (this may be due to failure of acetylcholine synthesis and hence really a pre-synaptic defect). The relationship to the thymus in myasthenia may be associated with the formation of antibodies against the neuromuscular junction. Myasthenia gravis may present clinically with double vision (diplopia), drooping eyelids (ptosis), a toneless voice or fatigue on chewing and swallowing. A myasthenic syndrome can occur in association with small-celled bronchial carcinoma, possibly due to interference with the release of acetylcholine from nerve terminals.

(iv) *Muscle membrane.*—Myotonia, a failure of the muscles to relax properly, is probably due to a disorder in the membrane of the muscle fibres. There are two main forms:

(*a*) dystrophia myotonia (autosomal dominant inheritance; myotonia, but in addition muscle dystrophy occurs often with E.C.G. disorders, and also cataracts and genital atrophy; recently disorders of smooth muscle have been reported, e.g. dysphagia);

(*b*) myotonia congenita (Thomsen's disease; inherited as an autosomal dominant; prolonged tonic contraction of muscles without wasting).

In addition, alteration of the relationship between potassium inside and outside the muscle cell (see Properties of Excitable Membranes, Chapter X) may lead to muscle weakness (commonest type is hypokalaemic familial periodic paralysis where there is a reduced plasma potassium level; in the hyperkalaemic form the plasma potassium is raised if severe but can be normal).

(v) *Disorders of the contractile machinery itself*, e.g. the muscular dystrophies, inflammatory myopathies (e.g. polymyositis, dermatomyositis). The muscular dystrophies are a group of genetically-determined degenerative disorders of muscle (the following six types are now generally recognised: Duchenne, limb-girdle, distal, facio-scapulo-humeral, ocular and congenital). Myopathies are also encountered due to carcinoma (particularly of breast, gastro-intestinal tract, bronchus, ovary). There may also be a defect in the supply of energy to the contractile machinery, a *metabolic myopathy*, e.g. McArdle's syndrome (where glycolysis of muscle glycogen is abnormal due to myophosphorylase deficiency; a similar disorder is due to muscle phosphofructokinase deficiency). Muscle damage can be produced by *chemical agents* (e.g. chloroquine, alcohol). There are various forms of *endocrine myopathy* (e.g. chronic thyrotoxic myopathy where there may be a disturbance in oxidative phosphorylation: see Chapter I; muscle degeneration may occur in Cushing's syndrome or with long-term steroid therapy, particularly when a fluorine atom is in the 9α-position: see Chapter II). The energy for contraction ultimately comes from the oxidation of carbohydrates and fatty acids (see Chapter I), but ATP provides the immediate energy for muscle contraction, while the ATP is regenerated from the high-energy phosphate linkage of creatine phosphate (creatine is re-phosphorylated from glycogen breakdown, both anaerobically and aerobically).

Chapter XII

BODY METABOLISM AND TEMPERATURE CONTROL

A DIET must contain sufficient quantities of the following for proper nutrition of the body:

> calories
> fat
> protein
> water
> minerals
> vitamins.

The metabolism of these materials in the body is often considered elsewhere (e.g. cell metabolism in Chapter I; water in Chapter IV; some vitamins in Chapter V), but the general requirements of man will be reviewed here.

Calories

Ingested food supplies the energy for growth, maintenance of vital functions and physical activity. The dietary sources of energy are carbohydrates, fats and proteins which on oxidation respectively produce 4·1, 9·3 and 4·1 kcals. per gram. They are utilized by cells to synthesise ATP (which is used as an energy source in chemical reactions in the body, see Chapter I) and the excess is lost as heat.

In the utilisation of these foodstuffs oxygen is utilised and carbon dioxide evolved (ratio of CO_2 evolution to O_2 consumption is the respiratory quotient, respectively 1·0 for carbohydrates, 0·80 for protein and 0·70 for fats). On usual diets the respiratory quotient is about 0·85, so the determination of the quantity of oxygen consumed will give a value for the heat produced in the body in that period. Heat production at rest is related to the surface area of the body, and is sometimes measured clinically from oxygen consumption twelve hours after a meal with the patient resting quietly (the basal metabolic rate).

Obesity occurs when intake of calories exceeds the output, the excess being converted to fat which is stored. Economic want or illness can cause insufficient calorie intake and weight loss followed by weakness and easy fatiguability (starvation).

Fats

When animal tissues are extracted by a non-polar ("fat") solvent a portion of the material may dissolve and this is known as *lipid*. This is a heterogenous group of substances whose principal members are:

(*a*) Simple lipids—esters of fatty acids with alcohols;
      triglycerides (esters of glycerol);
      waxes and glycerol ethers.
(*b*) Compound lipids—phospholipids (fatty acids, nitro-genous base, glycerol and phosphate);
      glycolipids (fatty acids, nitrogenous base, carbo-hydrate moiety).
(*c*) Derived lipids—fatty acids, sterols (e.g. cholesterol), fat-soluble vitamins.

In metabolism the term fats is considered to mean neutral lipids or triglycerides which are absorbed, after partial or complete hydrolysis, in the small intestine (see Chapter VII) and enter the blood as *chylomicrons*. The increase in chylomicrons in the blood after a meal produces turbid plasma and this can be "cleared" by lipoprotein lipase (released when heparin is injected). These absorbed triglycerides are metabolised to produce fatty acids which are used for the production of energy or else stored in the body in adipose tissue as triglyceride (the fatty acids stored as triglyceride are produced either from triglycerides transported in the blood or from acetyl-CoA in adipose tissue—see Chapter I).

The plasma lipids include triglycerides, phospholipid, cholesterol and free fatty acids (the latter are usually carried as an albumin complex, while the others are found in combination with specific globulins as lipoproteins which can be differentiated into low and high density fractions based on their characteristics during centrifugation). Plasma lipoprotein levels are affected by:

sex (males have higher levels of low density fraction than women until after menopause);

diet (especially dietary fat: unsaturated fat substituted for saturated fat, such as animal fat or hydrogenated oil, will reduce level of low density lipoproteins in plasma, e.g. cholesterol);

drugs (chlorphenoxyisobutyrate, or chlofibrate, reduces plasma cholesterol and triglyceride level).

Plasma free fatty acid (FFA) is derived from adipose tissue and breakdown of chylomicrons and is released when intracellular glucose is low and vice versa; glucose, insulin, tolbutamide, all cause a drop in circulatory FFA (due to decreased release). Plasma FFA is increased by the catecholamines (due to increased release from adipose tissue) and is raised in diabetic ketosis even with high blood glucose levels (for glucose is unable to enter cells properly in absence of insulin). FFA is a very important source of energy for the body's metabolism (e.g. supplies about 50 per cent energy for resting skeletal muscle).

CLINICAL DISORDERS OF LIPID METABOLISM

(a) Essential hyperlipaemia: rare: fasting plasma milky due to excess large lipoprotein molecules (particularly elevation triglyceride: sometimes hepatosplenomegaly or eruptive xanthoma): occasionally due to deficiency of heparin-induced lipoprotein lipase. In one similar form there are tuberose xanthomas.

(b) Essential hypercholesterolaemia with lipid deposited in extensor tendons, corneal arcus and xanthelasmas.

(c) Secondary hyperlipoproteinaemias, e.g. due to chronic biliary obstruction, nephrotic syndrome, myxoedema, diabetic ketosis.

(d) Hypolipoproteinaemias, e.g. absence of high density lipoproteins (Tangier disease), or syndrome of acanthocytosis and steatorrhoea recessively inherited.

There is a greater risk of developing coronary artery disease when plasma cholesterol levels are raised.

Proteins enter into the structure of all tissues, and the protein molecule is composed of large numbers of units called aminoacids. Ingested proteins are usually absorbed as amino-acids or small peptide chains and form body proteins while excess amino-acids are deaminated (NH_2 group broken off and excreted as urea) and either oxidized for energy or incorporated into other metabolic pathways (e.g. formation of glucose as in gluconeogenesis). When nitrogen loss (mainly in urine and faeces) is equal to nitrogen intake, nitrogen equilibrium exists, but increased intake is necessary for growth (and also in pregnancy) and also to replace loss of tissue protein, and in such a situation a positive nitrogen balance exists.

Although some amino-acids can be synthesised in the body (non-essential), at least ten are necessary preformed in the diet (essential, e.g. valine, leucine, phenylalanine, methionine, tryptophan, etc.) and should be present in about the proper proportions. Specific RNA molecules act as "templates" to line up the amino-acids and cause them to combine in the proper order for protein synthesis (see Chapter I).

Protein deficiency can occur due to poor diet (e.g. in southern U.S.A. and also in Africa where a form called Kwashiorkor is seen), chronic abscess, large burns, urinary leakage (e.g. nephrotic syndrome), and negative nitrogen balance is seen after operations and in bedridden patients. There are also disorders of protein synthesis (see Chapter V).

Water and mineral balance.—See Chapter IV (and Chapter II for Calcium Metabolism).

Vitamins are required in small amounts to catalyse certain body processes (often act as coenzymes to activate enzymes in metabolic processes). The early distinction made by McCollum and Davis is still used:

(i) fat-soluble (now composed of vitamins A, D, K);
(ii) water-soluble (includes vitamins B, C).

There are a number of substances, like pantothenic acid and biotin, which are presumed to be vitamins, whose role in human nutrition is unclear.

Vitamin A.—A lipid-soluble vitamin required for growth and development in children which, when deficient in the adult diet, causes xerophthalmia (desquamation and cornification of cornea and decreased lacrimation; "dry eye"), a dermatosis (perifollicular hyperkeratosis) and night blindness (the visual pigment rhodopsin is composed of a protein, opsin, and a carotenoid called retinene which is vitamin A aldehyde; see Chapter X). It is a higher alcohol stored mainly in the liver and the most potent source of supply is fish-liver oil.

Vitamin D.—The sterols vitamin D_2 (calciferol) and irradiated 7-dehydrocholesterol (vitamin D_3) and dihydrotachysterol all possess anti-rachitic activity. Vitamin D promotes intestinal absorption of calcium and calcification of the matrix of bone. Deficiency in children causes rickets and in adults leads to osteomalacia: this situation may arise from:

deficient diet (especially in growing children in association with lack of sunlight which irradiates the 7-dehydro-cholesterol in the skin, e.g. Pakistani children without supplementary milk or vitamins who live in industrial cities in the U.K.);

deficient absorption, e.g. intestinal malabsorption syndromes.

Hypervitaminosis D in children can occur due to excess intake or sensitivity to the vitamin with symptoms of hypercalcaemia (vomiting, polyuria and metastatic calcification, e.g. nephro-calcinosis).

Vitamin K.—Naphthoquinone derivatives necessary for the formation of prothrombin (see Chapter V), hence when deficient there is defective clotting of blood, e.g.:

due to defective absorption of vitamin K from the small intestine in obstructive jaundice;

due to defective formation of prothrombin from absorbed vitamin K in severe liver disease;

due to immaturity of prothrombin production mechanism in the liver in haemorrhagic disease of the newborn.

Vitamin B.—There are many factors in the vitamin B complex and their function will be summarised briefly below:

Thiamine is converted to the pyrophosphate by ATP and used in the oxidative decarboxylation of α-keto acids (e.g. oxaloacetic acid in the Krebs' cycle; see Chapter I).

Thiamine + ATP → thiamine pyrophosphate
Thiamine pyrophosphate + lipoic acid + coenzyme A
$$→ \text{acetyl-CoA} + CO_2$$
Acetyl-CoA + oxaloacetic acid → citric acid + coenzyme A.

A primary deficiency of thiamine can cause congestive heart failure and peripheral neuritis (see Chapter X).

Riboflavin.—Deficiency leads to cheilosis and seborrhoeic dermatitis about the nose, a magenta-coloured tongue and corneal vascularisation. In combination with nicotinamide and phosphate, it forms flavin adenine dinucleotide (FAD) which is an important enzyme in the mitochondrial electron transport chain concerned in carbohydrate metabolism (see Chapter I).

Nicotinic acid when deficient in the diet produces pellagra (characterised by dermatitis, diarrhoea and varying degrees of dementia; redness and soreness of the tongue is an early manifestation). It is involved in the electron transport chain (as the nicotinamide nucleotides, nicotinamide adenine dinucleotide or NAD and once called DPN, and nicotinamide adenine dinucleotide phosphate or NADP and once called TPN) (see Chapter I).

Pyridoxine (vitamin B_6) in the phosphate form is involved in transamination reactions, e.g. glutamine + α-keto acid by transamination will form α-amino acid. Deficiency in children can produce convulsions (seen when fed with a particular infant-feeding formula in the past) and also in a hypochromic anaemia which responds to an increased dietary intake of pyridoxine (not a true dietary deficiency); deficiency can be produced when isonicotinylhydrazide (isoniazid) is used to treat tuberculosis when a derivative of the drug competes with pyridoxal phosphate for certain sites on enzymes.

Biotin, choline and pantothenic acid have an unknown role in human metabolism at the present time.

Folic acid (as the tetrahydro derivative) is necessary as a carrier of hydroxymethyl and formyl groups and when deficient absorption occurs DNA synthesis is interfered with, producing a macrocytic anaemia and gastro-intestinal disturbances (see Chapter V).

Vitamin B_{12} is a porphyrin structure containing a cobalt atom and acts as a coenzyme in a series of apparently diverse reactions, although some involve the transfer of methyl groups (transmethylation).

Vitamin C.—Ascorbic acid is essential in man, primates and the guinea-pig but other species of animals can synthesise it. Its exact biochemical role is not clear although it has a role in producing tetrahydro-folic acid and also hydroxyproline formation which is necessary for collagen production. Deficiency produces scurvy with clinical manifestations due to functional failure of cells of mesenchymal origin (e.g. spongy gums with loose teeth, impaired capillary integrity with subcutaneous haemorrhages and epistaxis, a disturbance of growing bone affecting the osteoblasts and producing bone pain, lassitude and anorexia and anaemia; there is now considered to be failure of formation of normal connective tissue).

TEMPERATURE REGULATION

Internal body temperature is regulated in most vertebrates but in man there is a close control over this which can be understood better when the body is divided into:

(i) a central core of intrathoracic and intra-abdominal structures;

(ii) a peripheral shell of skin, subcutaneous tissue and muscle, and limbs.

Precise control of core temperature is maintained by permitting wide variations in temperature of the shell structures (the former is measured by a thermometer placed in the mouth or rectum), but for stabilization of core temperature heat gain must equal heat loss.

Heat gain.—This is measured by the basal (or better the sedated) metabolic rate mentioned earlier in this chapter, which can be altered by variation in thyroid hormone output (see Chapter II). Heat production can be increased by shivering and voluntary exercise; the initiation of shivering involves stimulation of receptors in the central nervous system and skin. Heat may be gained from the environment by radiation and conduction.

Heat loss.—Mostly by conduction, radiation and convection, and to a less extent by evaporation in temperate climates (but in tropical climates evaporation becomes more important). Coarse control is exercised by the amount and type of clothing worn and sweating, while fine control is mediated by adjusting the volume of blood flowing through the skin per minute (the latter depends on both peripheral and central temperature receptors with the latter probably being in the hypothalamus, while the former is a reflex event whose exact pathway is unknown). The rate of sweat production probably depends on both central and peripheral receptors. Local blood flow in the hand or foot can be varied by changing the temperature surrounding it, and for this a nerve supply is not needed so it possibly involves a direct action on the state of contraction of arterial smooth muscle.

Disorders of Temperature Regulation

These are seen in *fever* (abnormally high temperature) and in *hypothermia*.

An increased body temperature can be produced by injecting lipopolysaccharides extracted from certain bacteria and the bacterial pyrogen causes the liberation of a leucocyte pyrogen from white cells. In infectious fevers it is probably leucocyte antigen which acts on the central nervous system to upset its thermoregulatory functions possibly by an action on the hypothalamus to set the temperature regulatory mechanisms at an abnormally high threshold. Bacterial pyrogen is rapidly removed from the circulation by leucocytes and platelets, but probably does not produce the headache of fever by a direct action on pain-producing structures in the cranial cavity but rather via an intense vasoconstriction. Full explanations for the fever produced by prolonged heat exposure and familial periodic fevers await more work, although in the latter circulating steroids (e.g. unconjugated aetiocholanolone) may be involved.

Hypothermia results from reduced body heat production or abnormally high heat loss. The commonest causes in this country are:

neurological disorders, e.g. head injuries, cerebrovascular accidents, confusional states;

severe infections, e.g. bronchopneumonia;

endocrine disorders, e.g. myxoedema;

drugs affecting temperature regulation of the body, e.g. chlorpromazine, barbiturates, alcohol;

abnormal heat conservation mechanisms and haemodynamic abnormalities, e.g. loss of shivering response, postural hypotension.

REFERENCES

The following sources of reference were found most useful in compiling the book:

Chapter   I. *Principles of Biochemistry*, (3rd edit.), by White Handler and Smith.

General Pathology, (2nd edit.), by Walter and Israel.

Chapter   II. *Endocrinology* by Mason.

Chapter III. *Diseases of the Heart and Circulation*, (3rd edit.), by Wood.

Chapter IV. *Fundamentals of Acid-base Regulation*, (3rd edit.), by Robinson.

Chapter V. *Clinical Haematology in Medical Practice*, (2nd edit.), by de Gruchy.

Chapter VI. *Respiration* by Dejours.

Chapter VII. *Diseases of the Digestive System* by Truelove and Reynell.

Chapter VIII. *Diseases of the Digestive System* by Truelove and Reynell.

Chapter IX. *The Kidney*, (3rd edit.), by de Wardener.

Chapter X. *Clinical Neurology*, (2nd edit.), by Brain.

Chapter XI. *Clinical Neurology*, (2nd edit.), by Brain.

Constant reference was made to the series of *Handbooks of Physiology* produced by the American Physiological Society, the excellent textbook by Ruch and Patton, *Physiology and Biophysics*,(19th edit.), *Recent Advances in Medicine*, (14th and 15th edit.), by Baron, Compston and Dawson, and *Clinical Physiology* by Campbell and Dickinson acted as a form of "Pole Star" to guide me (a new edition of this book has appeared subsequently). Recourse was made on numerous occasions to the journals.

INDEX

Action potential, 138–141
Adenosine triphosphate, 5–7, 184
Adrenal, cortex, 20–24
  medulla, 24–25
Adrenocorticotrophic hormone, 12
Agranulocytosis, 76–77
Anaemia, 69–74
  due to blood loss, 69
  due to defective formation, 69–72
  due to increased destruction, 72–74
Androgenic steroids, 23
Antidiuretic hormone, 13
Apex cardiography, 41–42
Arrhythmias, cardiac, 35–36
Ascites, 120–121
Autonomic nervous system, 174–181
  higher control of, 179–181

Basal ganglia, 173–174
Bile, 117
Blood coagulation, 79–81
Blood gas
  carbon dioxide, 97–98
  oxygen, 96–97
  transport, 96–98
Blood glucose regulation, 27–28
Blood groups, 68–69
Blood vessels
  humoral control of, 50–51, 177–179
  nervous control of, 49–50
Body fluids, 61
Buffers, 22

Calcium metabolism, 19–20
Calories, 189–190
Carbon dioxide excretion, 94, 97–98
Cardiac muscle, 31–32
Cardiac output, 43–45
Cardiomyopathies, 32–33
Catecholamine metabolism, 179
Cell metabolism, 5–7
Cerebellum, 171–173
Cerebral circulation, 55–56
  cortex, 157–161
  occipital lobe, 160–161
  prefrontal lobe, 159–160
  sensory, 158–159
  temporal lobe, 160
Cerebrospinal fluid, 181–182
Chromosomal abnormalities, 3–4
Clearance, 123–124

Colon, 111–114
  abnormalities of function, 112–114
  assessment of function, 114
  movement, 114
Coma, 163
Compliance, 89
Consciousness, 162
Constipation, 112–113
Coronary circulation, 56
Corpus callosum, 161
Cyanosis, 98–99

Deafness, 169–170
Defaecation, 112
Deoxyribonucleic acid, 1–2
Depolarisation, 138–139
Diarrhoea, 113–114
Diffusion, 92
Diuretics, 131–132
Dwarfism, 11
Dysphagia, 102–103
Dyspnoea, 90

Ear, 168–171
  central auditory pathways, 169
Electrocardiography, 36–37
Electroencephalogram, 161
Emotion, 180–181
Eosinophilia, 77
Epilepsy, 161–162
Equilibration, 170–171
Erythropoietin, 26
Excitable membranes, properties of, 138–141
Extrapyramidal syndromes, 173–174
Eye, 163–168

Fat, dietary, 190–191
Fever, 196
Fibrinolytic system, 80–81
Folic acid, 70–72
Fundus oculi, 165–166

Gastric secretion, 103–105
  motility, 105–106
Gastrin, 103–104
Generator potential, 142–143
Glomerular function, 123
  impaired, 124–125

Glucocorticoids, 21–22
Glycogen storage disease, 115–116
Glycosuria, 125
Golgi apparatus, 1
Gonadotrophic hormones, 12, 28–30
Growth hormone, 11

Haemoglobin, 67, 72
  S, 73
Haemoglobinopathies, 73–74
Haemolysis, 72–74
Haemorrhagic disorders, 79–81
Haemostasis, 78
Hearing, 168–170
Heart sounds, 42–43
  failure, 45–48
  rate, 44
Hormones, 10–30
  adrenal cortex, 20–24
  adrenal medulla, 24–25
  anterior pituitary, 10–13
  gastrin, 103–104, 107
  kidney, 25–26
  ovary, 29–30
  pancreas, 27–28
  pancreozymin, 107
  parathyroid, 17–18
  pineal, 26
  placenta, 30
  posterior pituitary, 13
  secretin, 107
  testis, 28–29
  thymus, 26
  thyroid, 13–17
Hydrogen ion excretion, 59–61, 95
Hypertension, 51–52
  portal, 120
  pulmonary, 55
  systemic, 51–52
Hyperthyroidism, 15–16
Hypothalamus, 179–181
Hypothermia, 196
Hypothyroidism, 14–15
Hypoventilation, 90
Hypoxia, 94, 99–100

Immunoglobulins, 84–85
Intraocular fluid, 164–165
Ionising radiation, 7–9
Iron metabolism, 70

Jaundice, 118–120
Jugular venous pulse, 37–38
  abnormalities of, 38

Kidney
  anatomy, 122
  humoral function, 25–26
  physiology, 122–131

Left atrial pulse, 39
Leucocytes, 75–76
Leucytosis, 75–76
Leucopenia, 76
Leukaemia, 77
Lipids
  clinical disorders of, 191
  metabolism of, 190–191
Liver metabolism, 115–117
  function tests, 118
Lung volumes, 86–88

Malabsorption, 110–111
Metabolism, rate of, 189
Mineralocorticoids, 22–23
Mitochondria, 1, 5–7
Motoneurone lesions, upper, 152–153
  lower, 152–153
Murmurs, 38–40, 42
Muscle, 183–188
  contraction, 183–188
    clinical disorders of, 187–188
  mechanical performance, 186–187
  spindle, 143–144
  tone, 153–155
    clinical disorders of, 155–156

Nerves, humoral transmission of
    impulses, 177
  applied pharmacology of impulses,
    177–179
  vasomotor, 49–50
Neuromuscular function, 177–178,
    185–186
Neutropenia, 76–77
Nutrition, 189–195
Nystagmus, 168

Oedema, 65–66
Osteomalacia, 19
Osteoporosis, 19–20
Ovary, 29–30
Oxytocin, 13

Pacemakers, 33–35
Pancreas, 27–28
Parasympathetic nervous system, 175
Parathyroid glands, 17–18
Peripheral vascular system, 48–52
pH, 57–59
Phosphorus metabolism, 19–20
Pineal, 26
Pituitary gland, 10–13
Placental hormones, 30
Plasma, 81–85
  proteins, 82
  protein abnormalities, 83–85

Polycythaemia, 74–75
Portal hypertension, 120
Posture, 156–157
Potassium balance, 64–65
Prolactin, 12–13
Proteins, 191–192
Pulmonary circulation, 55
Pulse, arterial, 40–41
　venous, 37–39
Pupil, 163–164

Receptors, α and β, 50–51
Red cells, 67–69
　destruction, 68, 72–74
　formation, 68–72
　metabolism, 67–68
Reflex arc, 142, 145–148
　clinically important, 145, 147–148
　diminished tendon, 146
　flexor, 146–147
　stretch, 145
　tendon, 145
Refractory period, nerve, 140–141
Renal anatomy, 122
　clearance, 123–124
　disease, investigations in, 137
　failure, 134–137
　physiology, 122–131
　regulation of body pH, 130–131
　regulation of body Na^+, 131
　tubular defects, 132–134
　tubular function, 125–131
Renin, 25–26
Respiratory, function tests, 87–90
　failure, 100
Reticulo-endothelial system, 77–78
Rhesus factor, 68–69
Ribonucleic acid, 1–2
Ribosomes, 1–2

Saliva, 101
Sarcotubular system, 185–186
Secretin, 107
Sensation, clinical disturbances of, 150–151
Sensory receptors, 142–144

Shock, 53–54
Small intestinal digestion, 106–107
　absorption, 108–110
　assessment of function, 111
　disorders of absorption, 110–111
　disorders of secretion, 108
　secretion, 106–107
Sodium balance, 63–64
Spinal cord, organisation, 148–149
　ascending tracts, 148–149
　descending tracts, 152–153
Starling's law of the heart, 43–47, 186–187
　of the capillaries, 65
Stretch receptor, 143–144
Stroke volume, 43–44
Swallowing, 101–103
Sympathetic nervous system, 174–175

Temperature, regulation, 195
　disorders of regulation, 196
Testis, 28–29
Tetany, 17–18
Thrombocytopenia, 79
Thymus, 26
Thyrocalcitonin, 17
Thyroid, 13–17
Thyrotrophic stimulating hormone, 12

Ventilation, 86–96
　chemical control, 92, 94–95
　during muscle exercise, 96
　neural control, 92–94
　-perfusion ratio, 91
　regulating factors, 92–96
　uniformity of, 91
　utilisation of, 91–92
Vertigo, 171
Vision, 166–168
Visual fields, 166–168
Vitamins, 192–195
　B_{12}, 71, 110

Water balance, 63
White cells, 75–77